SLEEP AND ITS DISORDERS AFFECT SOCIETY

Edited by **Chris Idzikowski**

Sleep and its Disorders Affect Society
http://dx.doi.org/10.5772/56970
Edited by Chris Idzikowski

Contributors

Shinji Teramoto, Leila Azevedo, Fabiana Valera, Heidi Sander, Wilma Anselmo-Lima, Michelle A Miller, Carlos Zamarron, Carlos Rabade Castedo, Ester Zamarron De Lucas, Emilio Morete Aracay, Felix Del Campo, Marco Carotenuto, Maria Esposito, Rodrigo Iturriaga, Juan Idiaquez, Chris Idzikowski

Published by InTech

Janeza Trdine 9, 51000 Rijeka, Croatia

Publishing Process Manager Iva Lipovic

Technical Editor InTech DTP team

Cover InTech Design team

First published October, 2014

Printed in Croatia

Additional hard copies can be obtained from orders@intechopen.com

Sleep and its Disorders Affect Society, Edited by Chris Idzikowski

p. cm.

ISBN 978-953-51-1725-4

For EU product safety concerns:
IN TECH d.o.o., Prolaz Marije Krucifikse Kozulić 3, 51000 Rijeka, Croatia,
info@intechopen.com or visit our website at intechopen.com.

Meet the editor

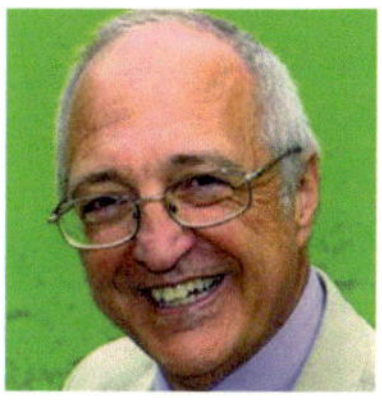

Dr Idzikowski's formal interest in sleep began in Edinburgh where he earned his PhD working with Emeritus Professor Ian Oswald, the UK's founding father of sleep research. He was Hon Treasurer of the British Sleep Society when it was first set up and subsequently became the founding Chairman of the Royal Society of Medicine Forum on sleep and its disorders and guided its transition to become the Sleep Medicine Section. He has held many honorary appointments, both health authority (Oxford) and University (e.g Queen's University of Belfast, Visiting Professor, Surrey University) and has also contributed to various sleep-related charitable organizations (e.g. Finland's Unettomat) as well as published numerous papers and books on sleep, including "Learn to sleep well" (Duncan Baird, 2000) and "Sleep" (Harper-Collins, 2007). Currently he is the Director of Edinburgh Sleep Centre, a Consultant Psychologist at the London Sleep Centre and the Director of Sleep Assessment and Advisory Service in Belfast.

Contents

Preface

I was delighted to be asked again by IntechOpen to edit another book for them on sleep. The books they publish have the enormous advantage of providing high quality, up to date information, mainly in a review format, in an Open Access setting. The sleep and sleep disorders area is rapidly expanding and has been so for many years now. When I started research into sleep, looking at sleep and memory specifically, the Pubmed database had 390 papers (against a background of 13,390 papers). Today, writing this preface there are now 5,304 papers on sleep and memory and 138,633 papers that mention sleep!

The association of sleep apnoea with cardiovascular, cerebrovascular and behavioural disorders and the various implications and ramifications demand continuing reviews of this area (1-7). Similarly, the impact of inadequate or restricted sleep on cognition continues to be both theoretically interesting but supremely important for the effects on the individual and society as a whole. My own chapter is more unusual and covers an emerging area, sleep-related sexual behaviours (a parasomnia - an unwanted or undesirable behaviour during sleep). On their own, they can have an effect on an individual or a relationship, but when this behaviour occurs in an inappropriate setting it can lead to substantial criminal retribution.

1. Jackman AR, Biggs SN, Walter LM, Embuldeniya US, Davey MJ, Nixon GM, et al. Sleep disordered breathing in early childhood: Quality of life for children and families. Sleep 2013, Nov;36(11):1639-46.

2. Tarasiuk A, Reuveni H. The economic impact of obstructive sleep apnea. Curr Opin Pulm Med 2013, Nov;19(6):639-44.

3. Bin YS, Marshall NS, Glozier N. The burden of insomnia on individual function and healthcare consumption in australia. Aust N Z J Public Health 2012, Oct;36(5):462-8.

4. Haaramo P, Rahkonen O, Hublin C, Laatikainen T, Lahelma E, Lallukka T. Insomnia symptoms and subsequent cardiovascular medication: A register-linked follow-up study among middle-aged employees. J Sleep Res 2014, Jun;23(3):281-9.

5. Moline M, DiBonaventura Md, Shah D, Ben-Joseph R. Impact of middle-of-the-night awakenings on health status, activity impairment, and costs. Nat Sci Sleep 2014;6:101-11.

6. Michal M, Wiltink J, Kirschner Y, Schneider A, Wild PS, Münzel T, et al. Complaints of sleep disturbances are associated with cardiovascular disease: Results from the gutenberg health study. PLoS One 2014;9(8):e104324.

7. Gilat H, Vinker S, Buda I, Soudry E, Shani M, Bachar G. Obstructive sleep apnea and cardiovascular comorbidities: A large epidemiologic study. Medicine (Baltimore) 2014, Jul;93(9):e45.

Chris Idzikowski
Innis Court, Holywood House,
Holywood, Co Down,
Northern Ireland BT18 9HF

Section 1

Sleep and Cognition

Chapter 1

Sleep and Cognition

Michelle A. Miller, Hayley Wright, Josie Hough and
Francesco P. Cappuccio

Additional information is available at the end of the chapter

http://dx.doi.org/10.5772/58735

1. Introduction

Sleep is an ancestral and primitive behaviour, an important part of life thought to be essential for restoration of body and mind. As adults, we spend approximately a third of our lives asleep and as we progress through life there are certain shifts in sleep architecture, most notably in sleep quantity. These biological or physiological age-dependent changes in sleep are well documented [1], and alongside the shifts in sleep architecture there is an increased susceptibility to certain sleep disorders.

Sleep disturbances and sleep deprivation are common in modern society. Most studies show that since the beginning of the century, populations have been subjected to a steady constant decline in the number of hours devoted to sleep. This is due to changes in a variety of environmental and social conditions (e.g. less dependence on daylight for most activities, extended shift work and 24/7 round-the-clock activities) [2].

Developments in the fields of molecular genetics, behavioural neuroscience, sleep neurobiology, and the cognitive neurosciences have produced converging evidence of a fundamental role for sleep in cognition. Sleep is required for good mental health, and insufficient sleep has negative effects on mood, cognitive performance and motor function [3]. Cognition is a broad term, which encompasses a variety of mental processes including memory, problem solving, language, forward planning and attention, which can all, be differentially affected by inadequate sleep. This can have serious real-life consequences, where many industries including airlines, long-distance truck driving, manufacturing and emergency services have recognised that sleep deprivation has major effects on performance.

Epidemiologists and clinical neuroscientists have also documented significant links between degree of sleep disturbance and severity of impairment on selective cognitive functions in a variety of clinical populations, including persons at risk for various dementing illnesses [4, 5].

Sleep disorder, in fact, may be one of the earliest signs of neurodegenerative disorders, including early Alzheimer's disease (AD) [6].

This chapter will briefly examine the relationship between sleep (quantity and quality) and cognition throughout the life course, and will consider the evidence which suggests that sleep deprivation and sleep disorders are associated with poor cognitive function. More specifically, it will examine the effects that sleep deprivation and sleep disorders have on both amnestic (memory function) and non-amnestic (non-memory function) cognitive processes.

2. Sleep quantity and cognition

Numerous studies have shown that short sleep, long sleep and sleep problems are associated with poorer cognitive function [7-9]. Self-reported short sleep, tiredness and fatigue are more strongly associated with subjective measures of cognitive function than with objective measures [7]. Findings from the Whitehall II study show that adverse changes in sleep over time (decrease from 6, 7 or 8 hours, or increase from 7 or 8 hours) are associated with lower scores on a variety of cognitive function tests, but not memory function [10]. Similarly, a Spanish study found that people who sleep for 11 hours or more per night have significantly lower global cognition scores than those who sleep for 7 hours [11]. A unique study has also reported on the effects of a post-lunch nap on subjective alertness and performance following partial sleep loss. A short nap has been found to improve alertness, sleepiness, short-term memory and accuracy, but does not affect reaction times [12].

Interestingly, there is little research into the effects of subtle changes in circadian phase on cognition, such as those that commonly occur in the general population after daylight saving time or returning to work after later weekend sleep. One study has revealed that performance on memory and verbal fluency tasks is significantly reduced on Monday morning following delayed weekend sleep [13]. Overall, proper alignment between sleep-wakefulness and internal circadian time may be crucial for cognitive performance, and humans may be very sensitive to small shifts in circadian timing.

The first recorded experiments on sleep deprivation began in the late 19th century [14], and research into the association between sleep and performance began around 50 years ago [15]. There is now clear evidence that deficits in daytime performance due to sleep loss are associated with a significant social, financial and human cost [3].

There are two types of sleep loss: acute sleep loss consisting of one continuous extended wake episode, and chronic sleep loss consisting of insufficient sleep over multiple days. A substantial amount of research has been conducted to understand the impact of short-term total sleep deprivation (<48h) on various cognitive domains. A recent meta-analysis examined the effect of sleep deprivation on six cognitive categories (simple attention, complex attention, working memory, processing speed, short-term memory and reasoning) for both speed and accuracy. Generally, effect sizes for each cognitive domain fall along a continuum, with tasks of greater complexity being less susceptible to the effects of total sleep deprivation. Simple attention, or vigilance, is most strongly affected by short-term sleep deprivation, emphasising that this deficit is the one for which compensation is least available. This has implications for tests of work fitness, where deficits in sustained attention could act as an early warning for subsequent cognitive failure in more complex situations [16].

Therefore, sleep debt can be expressed as an additional wakefulness that has a 'cost' (i.e. cognitive impairment), which accumulates over time [17]. Homeostatic physiological processes that occur during sleep can replenish this capacity, but how much sleep is required for satisfactory alertness and performance continues to be debated [18].

3. Sleep quality and cognition

Whereas sleep quantity is concerned with the amount of time we spend asleep, sleep quality is measured by how well we actually sleep during the night. This is usually assessed via self-reported frequency of nocturnal awakenings; difficulty initiating sleep; waking up early; or waking up feeling tired, using validated tools such as the PSQI [19]. Research has suggested that as well as sleep quantity, sleep quality may also play an important role in cognition. One such study in elderly women has found that disturbed sleep is associated with an increased risk of developing a cognitive impairment, but not with accelerated cognitive decline [20]. However, self-reported poor sleep is not independently related to cognitive function in community-dwelling older men, suggesting that there may be an interplay between sleep quantity and quality which accounts for the detrimental effects on cognitive function [21]. The Maastricht Ageing Study (MAAS) aimed to determine whether subjective sleep complaints (i.e. difficulty falling asleep, waking up too early, and restless or disturbed sleep) in middle aged and older adults predict global cognitive decline over a period of 3 years. The study found that subjective sleep complaints are negatively associated with cognitive performance at follow-up, where waking up too early has the strongest association with cognitive decline of the three sleep quality assessment questions [22]. However, the association between sleep complaints and cognitive decline disappears once depression is controlled for, raising the question of whether poor quality of sleep leads directly to poor cognitive function, or whether poor sleep causes an increase in depressive symptoms which then results in cognitive decline [22]. This finding highlights the importance of accounting for the effects of other variables, such as depression, on sleep and cognitive function when interpreting various study results and potentially contradictory conclusions.

4. Sleep and cognition: A life course perspective

The amount of time we spend asleep fluctuates across the lifespan according to changes associated with age, health and life events. Newborn infants need between 10.5 and 18 hours sleep per day, and this gradually reduces to between 9 and 12 hours by the end of the first year of life [23], before we settle into a pattern of around 7 to 8 hours sleep per night as adults [2].

Studies indicate that as we age, total sleep quantity, sleep efficiency and deep sleep tend to decline, whereas the incidence of waking after sleep onset tends to increase [24]. More specifically in terms of sleep architecture, the time spent in deep, slow wave sleep (SWS) diminishes, along with a decrease in rapid eye movement (REM) sleep, and the time spent in lighter, stage 1 and stage 2 sleep increases. As a consequence, older people often find it takes longer to fall asleep, have more fragmented sleep, and wake up earlier [1]. Furthermore, ageing is also associated with increased daytime sleep via napping and dozing. Gender and socioeconomic dynamics also play an important role during the life course in determining sleep patterns and their potential effect on health [25]. For example, in women, sleep is affected by life events such as pregnancy and the menopause. In the following sections, we consider the possible effects that these changes in sleeping patterns may have on cognitive function.

4.1. Sleep and cognition in childhood and adolescence

It is well established that sleep plays a vital role in brain maturation and in the development of important cognitive functions, such as memory consolidation and learning [26]. With modern advances in technology, many environmental factors and social activities potentially restrict the time spent sleeping once children and adolescents retire to the bedroom. For example, televisions, mobile phones and computers or video games are becoming common bedroom fixtures [27].

A typical child spends more time asleep than engaged in any other activity during the 24 hour cycle. As a rule of thumb, the optimal amount of sleep for children is more than 12 hours per night for pre-schoolers, about 12 hours per night for primary school children, and about 9 hours per night thereafter [26]. Between the ages of 3 and 5 years, there is a shift in sleep architecture, with a significant reduction in total sleep time and a decrease in the amount of time spent in 'deep' sleep, SWS and REM stages [28]. Further, sleep is distributed across the day until around the age of 5 years, when children shift from a polyphasic to a monophasic sleep pattern, usually due to the changes in daytime schedule associated with attending school [29]. It is commonplace for toddlers and pre-schoolers to engage in midday naps but, until recently, relatively little was known about the function and structure of this sleep period in children. Research has now shown that classroom naps consolidate learning in preschool children, and that the memory loss associated with nap-deprivation is not reversible with overnight sleep [30]. When children are allowed to nap during the day, they recall around 10% more learned material on waking than when tested after an equivalent period of being kept awake. Sleep spindle density in particular is strongly implicated in this memory consolidation process in children, highlighting that the nap does not merely protect the memory from wakeful interference, but that consolidation of learned material is a process unique to sleep [30]. This finding has implications for educational strategies, where scheduled classroom naps could enhance interventions designed to help children achieve academic goals and acquire necessary cognitive skills, with particular relevance to children with a learning delay [30].

There have been few longitudinal studies of sleep-wake patterns in children [31, 32], and only a small number of studies have investigated sleep behaviours [33, 34]. Therefore, what constitutes normal sleep patterns and normal sleep behaviour during childhood is still debatable. The lack of available data undoubtedly reflects the challenges to studying sleep in children and adolescents, which include reluctance of parents to leave children in the care of unfamiliar adults in laboratory studies, children's sleep becoming further disrupted in unfamiliar environments, and the potential for increased risk (e.g. fall in school performance, vehicle accidents in young drivers) following sleep restriction studies [35]. However, data from available studies has shown that sleep deprivation has a significant impact on cognitive abilities in children. Children aged between 10 to 14 years who are restricted to only 5 hours sleep show impaired cognitive performance on verbal creativity and the Wisconsin Card Sorting task, in comparison to those allowed to sleep for 11 hours [36]. Similarly, in a further study, children who are allowed to sleep for one hour longer perform significantly better in continuous performance and simple reaction time tests than those who sleep for one hour less, or those who receive no intervention [37]. Longitudinal research has shown that over the course of 3 years, children who experience an increase in sleepiness also show slower improvement in verbal comprehension than children who report lower levels of sleepiness at baseline [38]. The authors highlight the need for interventions to remedy sleep disorders and reduce the deleterious effect on cognition before the transition to puberty [38].

Circadian rhythms shift developmentally and sleep physiology changes considerably during adolescence (particularly SWS), which may alter the response to sleep restriction [39]. During the weekends, bed times and waking times can change extensively and persistently in children and in adolescents. These shifts are much more likely in adolescence, when the sleep phase rhythm can be seriously disrupted during weekends, and sleep debt is common [40]. Furthermore, the effects of delayed sleep phase in adolescents (characterised by problems with falling asleep and rising at appropriate times) extend into the week, where associations with lower average school grades, and greater incidence of anxiety and depression have been reported [41]. However, the effects of sleep duration on cognition can be different for males and females during the adolescent period. Whilst male adolescents who sleep for 8 hours or more demonstrate higher overall cognitive performance than those sleeping less than 8 hours, there is no association between sleep and cognition for adolescent females [42]. This supports previous findings that cognition is more susceptible to the effects of sleep deprivation in males than in females [43], and the authors propose that this is also consistent with the evolutionary demands of the female role in child rearing and nurturing [42].

4.2. Sleep and the elderly

Cognitive ageing is a heterogeneous process, in that not everyone experiences the same rate of decline. Indeed, many neuronal changes associated with cognitive decline begin to appear during middle-age [44]. Biological or physiological age-dependent changes in sleep have been well documented, and include shifts in sleep architecture as well as increased susceptibility to certain sleep disorders [1]. In addition to changes in SWS and REM, electroencephalography (EEG) studies have shown specific changes to delta waves, sleep spindles and K complexes during sleep in the elderly. It has been hypothesized that some of these changes might be early biological markers of the gradual deterioration of the central nervous system with age [45].

Furthermore, chronic ill-health, disability, and pain and discomfort at night may also contribute to poor sleep quality in an ageing population [46].

Ageing is associated with increased daytime sleep via napping and dozing, due to excessive daytime sleepiness (EDS) or feeling not rested upon awakening [47, 48]. The Medical Research Council Cognitive Function and Ageing Study (CFAS) looked at the association between self-reported sleep measures and cognition in over 2, 000 cognitively unimpaired individuals over the age of 65 years. The authors found that daytime napping at baseline is associated with a lower risk of cognitive decline at 2 and 10 year follow-ups, and that reports of both EDS and obtaining less than 6.5 hours of night-time sleep at baseline are associated with an increased risk of cognitive decline at 10 year follow-up [49]. Sleep structure is also important in aged adults, where the duration of sleep cycles, but not the amount of REM, non-REM or SWS or total sleep time, is positively associated with morning memory performance [50].

Sleep problems are a common occurrence in those with mild cognitive impairment (MCI) [51] and dementia [52]. Those with dementia experience highly fragmented sleep, with frequent daytime napping and night-time periods of wakefulness. Furthermore, sleep disorders have been associated with, and are predictive of, cognitive decline [5], and severity of cognitive impairment in diseases such as dementia and AD [53, 54]. A study has shown that non-demented, Japanese-American men who report EDS at baseline are twice as likely to be diagnosed with incident dementia at 3 year follow-up examination than those without EDS [55]. These findings were replicated in a sample of elderly French men and women [56], with the cross-cultural validation adding weight to the association between EDS and incident dementia.

Studies have also reported on sleep disturbances in specific types of dementia. In AD, for instance, which is characterized by episodic memory impairment, there are changes in global sleep architecture [57]. Modifications in the stages of sleep, including increased stage 1 sleep and reduced SWS, as well as decreases in sleep spindles, are well documented in dementia and AD [58, 59]. Less time in bed is associated with better cognitive function in AD [60], whereas EDS is strongly predictive of vascular dementia [61]. Changes in sleep architecture and sleep disturbances are found in a range of other neurodegenerative disorders such as progressive supranuclear palsy, Huntington's disease (HD), Parkinson's disease (PD), multiple system atrophy (MSA), dementia with Lewy bodies (DLB) and Creutzfeldt–Jakob disease (CJD) [57]. Only a few studies, however, have investigated the prospective association between sleep architecture and later neurodegenerative disorder. Furthermore, the available results are inconsistent, which may be due to population selection, duration of follow-up, age of participants or type of cognitive impairment [57].

4.3. Partum

Pregnant women experience prolonged sleep latency, frequent awakenings, fewer hours of night sleep, and reduced sleep efficiency, which begins in the second trimester of pregnancy and extends through at least the first 2-3 months after delivery [62, 63]. Sleep quality diminishes progressively throughout pregnancy, is most affected immediately after delivery, and then subsequently improves steadily [64]. Whilst many new mothers report feelings of confusion and forgetfulness during the early postpartum period, objective investigations thus far have not provided equivocal results. In some studies, women have significantly lower scores on tasks of immediate memory, complex mental functions (e.g. problem solving) and overall daytime function during the immediate postpartum period, with suggestions that this is influenced by sleep disturbance (e.g. fragmentation, deprivation) [62, 65, 66]. Indeed, although overall cognitive scores may not always differ between new mothers and controls, performance on memory and concentration tasks in postpartum women is significantly predicted by the amount of sleep they had the night before [63].

4.4. Menopause

Sleep complaints during or after menopause are a common medical problem. Whereas some studies have shown an association between sleepiness, sleep complaints and cognitive performance during and after menopause [67], other studies have not shown this association [68]. For example, one study showed that both self-reported and objectively-measured disturbed sleep are associated with diminished cognitive function during and after menopause. However, another study has showed that there is a higher association between self-reported poor sleep quality, rather than objectively measured poor sleep quality, and decreased cognitive test performance [69]. Weber et al found that memory complaints in particular are associated with increased sleep disturbance in perimenopausal women [70]. However, it has been suggested that it is age, rather than the menopause *per se*, which contributes to the decrease in cognitive performance [68].

5. Sleep disruption and work

Modern society depends on the continuous operation of a diverse array of crucial services. Thus the 24-hour culture-with shift work, night work, and longer, irregular working hours, and the associated shorter quantity of sleep-is becoming a frequent occurrence throughout the world [71, 72]. Sleep deprivation and consequent disruption of the circadian rhythm is a common situation experienced by individuals in many different professions, such as medical staff. After 8 hours of work, an individual's performance and ability to concentrate decreases, whilst the risk of fatigue [73] and cognitive errors increases [74]. Consequently, working at night and working excessive hours that restrict sleep opportunity are implicated in compromised health and safety at work [75]. A combination of factors are involved in this process including age, shift pattern, changes in sleep quality and quantity, sleep disruption and shorter daytime sleep (as compared to the usual night-time sleep), sleepiness and fatigue, and repeated stress induced by desynchronization of the circadian system [76, 77].

Sleepiness in the medical profession is a common occurrence due to the extensive hours worked and disturbed sleep [78]. During a typical shift, physicians perform complex problem solving whilst undertaking a multitude of different tasks. There is extensive research into the effects of sleep deprivation on specific tasks (such as endotracheal intubation and catheterization) [79], and in many different specialties such as anaesthetics [80], emergency medicine

[81], surgery or intensive care [82]. A landmark study of medical residents working in an adult intensive care unit shows that residents make more medical errors when they work frequent shifts of at least 24 hours, than when they work shorter shifts [83]. Thus, the effect of sleep deprivation on physicians could have a direct impact on quality of health care.

Subjectively, medical residents report disturbances of sleep, alertness and mood during the night float rotation [84]. Studies have also shown that residents are more likely to have a motor vehicle crash or 'near miss' after a night of on-call duty [85], or after a shift lasting 24 hours or longer [86]. Sleep-deprived residents also have more attention lapses, experience more adverse events and make more diagnostic errors while on duty overnight [86, 87]. From a training perspective, sleep deprivation may affect residents' skill acquisition and retention.

Aviators and aviation crews are also at a profound risk of sleep deprivation and disturbance given the nature and requirements of their work. Military pilots are required to synthesize vast amounts of information and subsequently make critical decisions. Thus, factors, which may impair cognitive performance, such as fatigue and sleep disruption, must be identified and alleviated wherever possible. A survey of US Army aircrew found that almost 62% of respondents did not feel that they received adequate daytime sleep while on shift [88]. A further study showed that there is a significant positive association between level of effectiveness (as determined by sleep–wake patterns) and neurocognitive functioning before flight operations [89]. In addition, the influence of chronic jet lag on cognitive efficiency in cabin crew has been investigated. Prolonged cortisol elevations (over 8 hours jet lag per week, for more than 3 years) results in a reduced temporal lobe volume within the brain, as well as deficits in spatial learning and memory, which become apparent after just five years of exposure to high cortisol levels [90].

Alongside studies into the effects of shift work and subsequent sleep disruptions on cognitive function, there has been on-going research into performance enhancers for shift and night workers. Various studies have found that improvements in alertness and performance during night shifts are associated with the use of stimulants such as caffeine [91] and modafinil [92, 93], and even exposure to bright light [94]. Laboratory and field studies corroborate that scheduled exposure to bright light (for work) and darkness (for sleep) shifts the circadian clock to align completely with a night work/day sleep schedule [95, 96]. As mentioned previously regarding post-lunch naps [12], short naps may also be useful for improving alertness during night shifts [91]. However, these countermeasures do not address the underlying cause of the problem, which is misalignment between circadian rhythms and the sleep and work schedule.

Few studies have assessed the *long-term* consequences of chronic sleep deprivation and repeated disruption of circadian rhythms on cognitive function. Findings from the Whitehall II study show that working more than 55 hours per week is associated with short sleep and lower scores in many cognitive performance tests, including vocabulary and reasoning, at both baseline and 5 year follow-up [97]. Another key study has found that male shift workers have lower cognitive scores and slower cognitive processing than those who have never been exposed to shift work, and that memory performance decreases with increasing shift-work duration [98]. Interestingly, individuals who ceased shift work more than 4 years earlier demonstrated no cognitive impairments, which suggest that the effect of shift work on cognitive function may be reversible [98]. Overall, these results imply that long term exposure to shift work, resulting in insufficient sleep due to a disrupted circadian rhythm, leads to the deterioration of cognitive function (at least in men).

6. Sleep and amnestic and non-amnestic cognition

The term 'cognition' refers to various higher mental processes, which allow us to think, perceive, remember, imagine and plan ahead in everyday life. These specific processes can be grouped into two broader categories of 'amnestic' (memory) and non-amnestic (not involving memory) cognitive function. This is a useful dichotomy when considering age-related cognitive decline and the conversion from normal cognitive ageing to MCI, since MCI is typically diagnosed as amnestic (aMCI) or non-amnestic (naMCI) type [99]. These two types of MCI have different trajectories, with aMCI potentially developing into AD, and naMCI possibly developing into various forms of dementia (e.g. vascular dementia, DLB, frontotemporal dementia) [100].

Despite the advance in knowledge of MCI subtypes, to date, most studies into the effects of sleep on cognitive function have reported results from tests of 'global' cognitive function, such as the Mini-Mental State Exam (MMSE) [101]. Nevertheless, it is possible to distinguish between amnestic and non-amnestic function using the MMSE, as reported recently in a study on sleep characteristics and subsequent cognitive impairment at one-year follow up [102]. In this study, amnestic cognitive impairment is distinguished from non-amnestic impairment by scores on the delayed recall task in the MMSE. That is, if participants cannot recall any of the three items in the memory task, or can only recall one of the items, this is categorised as a failure and thus the participant is attributed with an amnestic cognitive impairment. With regards to sleep quantity, amnestic cognitive impairments at one-year follow up are significantly predicted by long sleep durations (≥ 9 hours) in women, and by short sleep durations (≤ 5 hours) in men. It is possible that women are more resilient to the effects of short sleep due to environmental demands [42], or that men are more susceptible than women to cognitive impairment following sleep deprivation [43], although the authors urge that sex differences in these results should in interpreted with caution [102]. That is, males made up a smaller proportion of the sample and so some effects may not be detected due to a lack of statistical power. In addition, there was no association between sleep quantity and non-amnestic function in this sample of community-dwelling older adults.

Gaining knowledge of different predictors of amnestic and non-amnestic cognitive impairment is important, now more than ever, owing to the advances in MCI and dementia research which will eventually allow earlier, and more accurate, diagnoses of cognitive impairments and dementia. Although Potvin et al. (2012) have shown that the MMSE can be used to extract amnestic and non-amnestic cognitive scores; the findings should be interpreted with caution [102]. Relying on the results of one item from a test of global cognition is not a robust method of diagnosing memory impairment, not merely because there are so many more tests, which comprise the non-amnestic score on the MMSE. Further research is now needed to validate and standardise specific tests of amnestic and non-amnestic cognitive function, which will allow more accurate and specific diagnoses of MCI subtypes, thus giving way to earlier detection and diagnoses of dementia and AD, which in turn will improve the level of support provided to patients and their families.

7. Sleep disordered breathing, sleep disorders and cognitive function

The term sleep-disordered breathing (SDB) refers to conditions, which are characterised by intermittent reduction (hypopnoea) or cessation (apnoea) of breathing due to narrowing of the upper airways. These apnoeas and hypopnoeas occur during sleep, causing recurrent arousals from sleep and subsequent EDS. The condition is very common in the elderly, with reports of prevalence rates between 24 and 42% [103]. Each of the two consequences of SDB (sleep fragmentation and hypoxia) is associated with the risk of developing neurocognitive impairments in various domains [5, 104, 105].

7.1. Sleep apnoea

The most common form of sleep apnoea is obstructive sleep apnoea (OSA) or obstructive sleep apnoea syndrome (OSAS). OSAS is associated with frontal lobe and subcortical damage, which in turn is associated with diminished attention span, memory, delayed recall, impaired language and executive functions [106]. Research suggests that the specific brain damage associated with OSAS could therefore increase the risk of developing dementia [107]. Furthermore, a significant positive correlation between the apnoea index (the number of apnoeas occurring per hour) and severity of dementia has also been reported in AD patients [108]. Indeed, SDB may exacerbate cognitive dysfunction in patients with dementia and AD [109].

The EDS associated with OSAS usually becomes worse as AD progresses. Several studies have suggested a relationship of EDS with the occurrence of dementia [55, 56, 61], but it remains unclear as to whether SDB precedes cognitive impairment or vice versa. It is imperative that the causal associations are established as SDB has a high rate of associated morbidity, and utilisation of established and effective treatments (such as continuous positive airways pressure (CPAP)) might prevent or slow future cognitive decline. For instance, research has shown that treatment of OSA via CPAP improves some aspects of cognitive function in dementia patients as well as in non-demented elderly patients with OSA [109, 110]. However some neurobehavioural deficits, such as impairments in driving performance, may not be reversed by CPAP treatment in patients with severe OSA, and so further research is needed to assess the causes of such impairments [111].

7.2. Rapid eye movement sleep behaviour disorder (RBD)

RBD is a parasomnia, which is characterized by recurrent dream enactment and loss of normal voluntary muscle atonia during REM sleep, causing excessive motor activity [112]. These movements can cause excessive limb or body jerking leading to complex violent behaviours.

RBD is now recognized to be a symptom or prodrome of the group of diseases, which include PD, MSA and DLB [113]. The first study to document this relationship reported that 38% of patients diagnosed with isolated, idiopathic RBD later went on to develop a Parkinsonian disorder after a mean of 12.7 years from RBD onset [114]. Subsequent studies have confirmed similar findings, with typical mean intervals from RBD to PD, DLB, or MSA of around a decade [115-117]. This lengthy preclinical phase has important implications for interventions, which are designed to slow or halt the neurodegenerative process [4], and could therefore potentially slow the rate of associated cognitive decline.

7.3. Insomnia

Insomnia is a commonly reported sleep disorder in Western European countries. It is estimated that between 10% and 35% of the population of Western Europe have varying degrees of insomnia symptoms [118]. Insomnia has been defined in a variety of different ways in epidemiological research, from the presence of any difficulty initiating or maintaining sleep through to validated diagnostic criteria provided by the Diagnostic and Statistical Manual of Mental Disorders [119], with prevalence rates varying with each definition [120].

There is a growing amount of literature showing that insomniacs are at increased risk of cognitive decline (see [121] for a review). One study has shown that insomniacs have decreased memory ability compared to normal sleepers, where the detrimental performance is not attributable to sleepiness [122]. Furthermore, performance deficits in reaction times and vigilance tests often found in insomniacs may be related to specific SWS deficiencies [123].

8. Mechanisms

The underlying mechanisms regarding the association between sleep and cognition are still relatively poorly understood. However, specific brain regions involved with certain neuro-cognitive domains, including executive attention, working memory and higher cognitive functions, are known to be particularly vulnerable to sleep deprivation [3]. Furthermore, it has been suggested [124] that fragmented daytime sleep (following a night shift) is associated with large reductions in activity in the corticothalamic network, which mediates alertness, attention and higher-order cognitive processes. Performing higher-order cognitive tasks, such as decision-making, at night may be reliant on prefrontal brain areas, which suggests either the recruitment of a focused attentional strategy, cortical compensation for sleep deprivation, or both [125].

Despite decades of research, the significance and functions of sleep and its various stages, in particular REM sleep, are still not fully understood. A close association with cognitive functions was assumed shortly after the discovery of REM sleep and its relationship to dreaming [126] and there is now considerable evidence showing that newly learned material and skills are consolidated during REM sleep [127]. Furthermore, studies show a link between brain cholinergic activity, timing and density of REM sleep and cognitive functioning [128]. Thus, deficiencies of REM sleep might correlate with or predict cognitive deficits in the elderly.

Research linking SWS to mental restorative processes has been somewhat limited and less convincing. Only a few studies have attempted to examine the relationship between nocturnal SWS and subsequent daytime performance. In one study of healthy young male subjects, those who had slower reaction times on a daytime vigilance test also had lower amounts of nocturnal SWS than did age-and gender-matched individuals who had relatively faster reaction times [129]. Further to findings of the importance of SWS to daytime performance in younger people, Spiegel et al. report both confirmatory and contradictory results concerning the associations between loss of SWS and cognitive decline in adult life. They speculate that the role or functional significance of SWS may change over the course of the life span, which could account for their inconsistent findings, where SWS plays a restorative role in the cognitive functioning of older adults [130]. It is however possible that these studies are measuring different aspects of SWS and that the observed differences may reflect a lack of resolution in the available measurements.

The formation of long-term memories requires a process of consolidation, which is facilitated by sleep. The formation of declarative (consciously recalled) memories, which are hippocampus-dependent, appears to benefit mainly from SWS [131]. Recently, the focus has also been placed on stage 2 sleep and more precisely on sleep spindles, where research shows that overnight verbal memory retention is highly correlated with an increase in the number of sleep spindles [132].

Substantial inter-individual differences in vulnerability to the effects of sleep loss have been demonstrated by various studies [133]. These differences are partly due to tolerance of disturbances in circadian and social rhythm, which varies considerably between individuals [134]. There is also substantial individual variability in the magnitude of age-related cognitive decline [135]. Suggested sources for this variability focus on individual differences in the amount of age associated brain dysfunction, such as cortical [136], white matter pathology [137], and reductions in neurotransmitter receptor binding [138].

Sleep deprivation, mental fatigue, depression, or sleep disorders such as narcolepsy may result in an individual experiencing a transient loss of perception of external stimuli. This is known as a microsleep, and may last up to 30 seconds [139]. Microsleeps can occur at any time without warning, and the sufferer is usually unaware of the occurrence. As such, microsleeps are extremely dangerous in situations that require constant attention or vigilance, such as driving or operating heavy machinery [140]. Through a combination of EEG and neuroimaging techniques, research has shown that there are distinct and localised increases in activity in the fronto-parietal cortex which accompany microsleeps [141]. This activity may be part of a mechanism to restore responsiveness during the transient loss of arousal. Positron Emission Tomography (PET) studies have also confirmed that the 'resting brain' is surprisingly active. Raichle and Mintun (2006) report that, not only are there specific areas of the brain associated with higher regional cerebral blood flow (rCBF) during rest than during attention-demanding tasks, but that attention-demanding tasks are associated with just a 10% increase in global brain metabolism compared to periods of rest [142]. The Default Mode Network (DMN) is responsible for the default state of 'resting' brain activity, which is vital for brain functioning and possibly consciousness [143]. The DMN comprises the posterior and anterior cingulate cortex, and the temporo-parietal cortex [144], where activity decreases during attention-demanding tasks and increases when no such tasks are preformed (i.e. during rest) [145]. Interestingly, Picchioni et al. (2008) also found a transient increase in activity within the DMN during early stage 1 sleep [146].

Closely related to the DMN is the process of 'mind wandering' (or daydreaming), which is described as the default mode of operation of the brain [144]. It has been argued that rather than being a passive process, mind wandering is vital to healthy cognition, for example by integrating past and present experiences to facilitate future planning and personal goal resolution [147]. There has been speculation regarding the similarity between thought processes involved in mind wandering during wakeful periods and dream mentation during sleep [148], encouraging a more scientific enquiry into whether daydreaming and dreaming are mediated by the same neural networks. Indeed, meta-analyses of neuroimaging data show overlaps in activation of areas of the DMN during mind wandering, and dreaming during REM sleep [148].

9. Public health importance

There is no doubt that sleep is an integral part of life, and many studies have suggested that it should not be overlooked by clinicians, especially in older adults. Studies have shown that poor sleep quality can be an early sign of amnestic cognitive decline [102] and that EDS may be an early marker and potentially reversible risk factor of cognitive decline and onset of dementia [56].

Cognitive failures associated with total sleep deprivation are of great interest and importance, as their real-world consequences are often catastrophic [149, 150]. Night work is associated with safety risks for both the individual worker as well as society [149, 151]. Deficits in many aspects of cognition such as decision-making, memory processes and importantly in sustained attention are implicated in errors and accidents [16]. Diminished alertness during night shifts has been linked to ability to drive a motor vehicle, which can result in accidents [80, 85, 152]. There is also evidence that air traffic controller (ATC) performance declines and error rates increase on the night-shift, and that ATCs may be falling asleep while on-duty [153]. This, together with the evidence that flying performance decrements occur due to fatigue [154], poses a real worry. Considerable controversy exists regarding optimal work hours for physicians and surgeons, especially those in training [86]. There is a trade-off between providing a continuity of care; educational opportunities; and traditionally defined professionalism vs. clinicians' fatigue and health; erroneous decision-making and performance; patient care and safety; and overall cost of health care [152, 155].

The implementation of the European Working Time Directive (EWTD) has dramatically shortened doctors' working hours in an effort to reduce resident fatigue, with the anticipated result of decreasing fatigue-related medical errors and improving residents' well-being

[156]. Following the implementation of these regulations, increasing attention has been focused on the role of resident physicians' fatigue and the occurrence of medical errors, percutaneous needle sticks, laceration injuries and post-call motor vehicle crashes [157]. Although certain aspects remain controversial, there seems to be a positive effect on residents' fatigue levels, quality of life and job satisfaction, which may positively influence patient safety [158, 159]. Despite these changes, long working hours remain a common feature in health care worldwide [160]. An evidence-based approach is needed to minimize the risk that current work hour practices bestow while optimizing education and continuity of care [86].

Research shows that the effect of sleep deprivation on cognition is an important public health issue. Results of these studies have important implications in many areas of society, from new policies in medical education [87] to flight psychologists, improving overall sleep patterns and enhancing the war-fighting efforts of aviators in combat [89]. Understanding the fundamental properties and mechanisms through which sleep disruption and sleep disorders are related to cognition, and how sleep regulates alertness and performance in humans, also has therapeutic implications for the development of treatment and prevention strategies, as well as novel wake-promoting therapies [18].

10. Conclusions

Studies to date suggest that sufficient quantity and quality of sleep are required for many aspects of amnestic and non-amnestic cognition, most notably executive attention, working memory and higher cognitive functions. The amount of sleep required continues to be debated, but it is generally agreed that people at the extremes of the sleep distribution, i.e. short (<5hr) and long (>9hr) sleepers [20], are subject to cognitive deficits and accelerated cognitive ageing. Proper alignment between sleep-wakefulness and internal circadian time is crucial for optimal cognitive performance.

A vast amount of research has been conducted into the effect of sleep on cognition in specific scenarios as highlighted in this review. Shift workers who may have shortened sleep patterns have been implicated in compromised health and safety at work due to cognitive deficits. Furthermore, during pregnancy, postpartum and the menopause, women are vulnerable to sleep disturbances, which can have profound effects on different areas of cognition, most notably memory. Age-dependent changes in sleep have been well documented, and research has been conducted into the association between these changes and effects on normal and pathological cognitive decline. Sleep disorders have also been shown to negatively affect cognitive function across the lifespan.

Further research is required to understand the associations and mechanisms involved in more detail, where the findings could have huge impacts in many areas of medicine, from normal ageing to neurocognitive disorders and public health.

Acknowledgements

The study is part of the *Sleep, Health & Society* Programme of The University of Warwick. This project was supported by a small grant from the University of Warwick Undergraduate Research Scholarship Scheme (URSS). We thank Patricia McCabe for help with the preparation of the manuscript.

Author details

Michelle A. Miller*, Hayley Wright, Josie Hough and Francesco P. Cappuccio

*Address all correspondence to: Michelle.miller@warwick.ac.uk

University of Warwick, Warwick Medical School, Coventry, UK

References

[1] Bliwise DL. Normal aging. Principles and practice of sleep medicine. Forth ed. Philadelphia: WB Saunders Company; 2005. p. 24-38.

[2] Cappuccio FP, Miller MA, Lockley SW. Sleep, health, and society: the contribution of epidemiology. In: Cappuccio FP, Miller MA, Lockley SW, editors. Sleep, Health, and Society: From Aetiology to Public Health. 1 ed. Oxford: OUP; 2010. p. 1-8.

[3] Durmer JS, Dinges DF. Neurocognitive consequences of sleep deprivation. Semin Neurol 2005;25(01):117-29.

[4] Claassen DO, Josephs KA, Ahlskog JE, Silber MH, Tippmann-Peikert M, Boeve BF. REM sleep behavior disorder preceding other aspects of synucleinopathies by up to half a century. Neurology 2010;75(6):494-9.

[5] Yaffe K, Laffan AM, Harrison SL, Redline S, Spira AP, Ensrud KE, et al. Sleep-disordered breathing, hypoxia, and risk of mild cognitive impairment and dementia in older women. JAMA: The Journal of the American Medical Association 2011;306(6): 613-9.

[6] Rauchs GA, Schabus M, Parapatics S, Bertran Fo, Clochon P, Hot P, et al. Is there a link between sleep changes and memory in Alzheimer's disease? Neuroreport 2008;19(11):1159-62.

[7] Kronholm E, Sallinen M, Suutama T, Sulkava R, Era P, Partonen T. Self-reported sleep duration and cognitive functioning in the general population. Journal of Sleep Research 2009;18(4):436-46.

[8] Nebes RD, Buysse DJ, Halligan EM, Houck PR, Monk TH. Self-reported sleep quality predicts poor cognitive performance in healthy older adults. The Journals of Gerontology Series B: Psychological Sciences and Social Sciences 2009;64(2):180-7.

[9] Xu L, Jiang CQ, Lam TH, Liu B, Jin YL, Zhu T, et al. Short or long sleep duration is associated with memory impairment in older Chinese: the Guangzhou Biobank Cohort Study. Sleep 2011;34(5):575-80.

[10] Ferrie JE, Shipley MJ, Akbaraly TN, Marmot MG, Kivimaki M, Singh-Manoux A. Change in sleep duration and cognitive function: findings from the Whitehall II Study. Sleep 2011;34(5):565-73.

[11] Faubel R, Lopez-Garcia E, Guallar-Castillon P, Graciani A, Banegas JR, Rodriguez-Artalego F. Usual sleep duration and cognitive function in older adults in Spain. Journal of Sleep Research 2009;18(4):427-35.

[12] Waterhouse J, Atkinson G, Edwards B, Reilly T. The role of a short post-lunch nap in improving cognitive, motor, and sprint performance in participants with partial sleep deprivation. Journal of Sports Sciences 2007;25(14):1557-66.

[13] Yang CM, Spielman AJ. The effect of a delayed weekend sleep pattern on sleep and morning functioning. Psychology and Health 2001;16(6):715-25.

[14] Patrick GTW, Gilbert JA. Studies from the psychological laboratory of the University of Iowa: On the effects of loss of sleep. Psychological Review 1896;3(5):469-83.

[15] Wilkinson RT. Interaction of lack of sleep with knowledge of results, repeated testing, and individual differences. J Exp Psychol 1961;62:263-71.

[16] Lim J, Dinges DF. A meta-analysis of the impact of short-term sleep deprivation on cognitive variables. Psychological Bulletin 2010;136(3):375-89.

[17] Van Dongen HP, Maislin G, Mullington JM, Dinges DF. The cumulative cost of additional wakefulness: dose-response effects on neurobehavioral functions and sleep physiology from chronic sleep restriction and total sleep deprivation. Sleep 2003 Mar 15;26(2):117-26.

[18] Cohen DA, Wang W, Wyatt JK, Kronauer RE, Dijk DJ, Czeisler CA, et al. Uncovering residual effects of chronic sleep loss on human performance. Science Translational Medicine 2010;2(14):14ra3.

[19] Buysse DJ, Reynolds CF 3rd, Monk TH, Berman SR, Kupfer DJ. The Pittsburgh Sleep Quality Index: a new instrument for psychiatric practice and research. Psychiatry Res 1989 May;28(2):193-213.

[20] Tworoger SS, Lee S, Schernhammer ES, Grodstein F. The association of self-reported sleep duration, difficulty sleeping, and snoring with cognitive function in older women. Alzheimer Dis Assoc Disord 2006;20(1):41-8.

[21] Blackwell T, Yaffe K, Ancoli-Israel S, Redline S, Ensrud KE, Stefanick ML, et al. Association of sleep characteristics and cognition in older community-dwelling men: the MrOS sleep study. Sleep 2011 Oct;34(10):1347-56.

[22] Jelicic M, Bosma H, Ponds RWHM, Van Boxtel MPJ, Houx PJ, Jolles J. Subjective sleep problems in later life as predictors of cognitive decline. Report from the Maastricht Ageing Study (MAAS). International Journal of Geriatric Psychiatry 2002;17(1): 73-7.

[23] National Sleep Foundation. How Much Sleep Do We Really Need? 2013. 30-6-2013.

[24] Bixler E. Sleep and society: an epidemiological perspective. Sleep Med 2009 Sep;10 Suppl 1:S3-S6.

[25] Hislop J, Arber S. Sleep, Gender, and Aging. In: Calsanti TM, Selvin KL, editors. Age Matters: Re-Aligning Feminist Thinking.New York: Routledge; 2006. p. 225-46.

[26] Spruyt K, Gozal D. Sleep in children: the evolving challenge of catching enough and quality Zzz's. In: Cappuccio FP, Miller MA, Lockley SW, editors. Sleep, Health and Society: From Aetiology to Public Health. 1st ed. Oxford: OUP; 2010. p. 215-38.

[27] Li S, Jin X, Wu S, Jiang F, Yan C, Shen X. The impact of media use on sleep patterns and sleep disorders among school-aged children in China. Sleep 2007 Mar;30(3): 361-7.

[28] Ohayon MM, Carskadon MA, Guilleminault C, Vitiello MV. Meta-analysis of quantitative sleep parameters from childhood to old age in healthy individuals: developing normative sleep values across the human lifespan. Sleep 2004 Nov 1;27(7):1255-73.

[29] Weissbluth M. Naps in children: 6 months-7 years. Sleep 1995 Feb;18(2):82-7.

[30] Kurdziel L, Duclos K, Spencer RMC. Sleep spindles in midday naps enhance learning in preschool children. Proc Natl Acad Sci USA2013 Oct 22;110(43):17267-72.

[31] Thorleifsdottir B, Bjornsson JK, Benediktsdottir B, Gislason T, Kristbjarnarson H. Sleep and sleep habits from childhood to young adulthood over a 10-year period. J Psychosom Res 2002 Jul;53(1):529-37.

[32] Iglowstein I, Jenni OG, Molinari L, Largo RH. Sleep duration from infancy to adolescence: reference values and generational trends. Pediatrics 2003 Feb;111(2):302-7.

[33] Iglowstein I, Latal HB, Molinari L, Largo RH, Jenni OG. Sleep behaviour in preterm children from birth to age 10 years: a longitudinal study. Acta Paediatr 2006 Dec; 95(12):1691-3.

[34] Jenni OG, Fuhrer HZ, Iglowstein I, Molinari L, Largo RH. A longitudinal study of bed sharing and sleep problems among Swiss children in the first 10 years of life. Pediatrics 2005 Jan;115(1 Suppl):233-40.

[35] Beebe DW. Cognitive, behavioral, and functional consequences of inadequate sleep in children and adolescents. Pediatr Clin North Am 2011 Jun;58(3):649-65.

[36] Randazzo AC, Muehlbach MJ, Schweitzer PK, Walsh JK. Cognitive function following acute sleep restriction in children ages 10-14. Sleep 1998 Dec 15;21(8):861-8.

[37] Sadeh A, Gruber R, Raviv A. The effects of sleep restriction and extension on school-age children: what a difference an hour makes. Child Dev 2003 Mar;74(2):444-55.

[38] Bub KL, Buckhalt JA, El-Sheikh M. Children's sleep and cognitive performance: a cross-domain analysis of change over time. Dev Psychol 2011 Nov;47(6):1504-14.

[39] Campbell IG, Higgins LM, Trinidad JM, Richardson P, Feinberg I. The increase in longitudinally measured sleepiness across adolescence is related to the maturational decline in low-frequency EEG power. Sleep 2007 Dec;30(12):1677-87.

[40] Crowley SJ, Acebo C, Carskadon MA. Sleep, circadian rhythms, and delayed phase in adolescence. Sleep Med 2007 Sep;8(6):602-12.

[41] Saxvig IW, Pallesen S, Wilhelmsen-Langeland A, Molde H, Bjorvatn B. Prevalence and correlates of delayed sleep phase in high school students. Sleep Med 2012 Feb; 13(2):193-9.

[42] Ortega FB, Ruiz JR, Castillo R, Chillon P, Labayen I, Martinez-Gomez D, et al. Sleep duration and cognitive performance in adolescence. The AVENA study. Acta Paediatr 2010 Mar;99(3):454-6.

[43] Alhola P, Polo-Kantola P. Sleep deprivation: Impact on cognitive performance. Neuropsychiatr Dis Treat 2007;3(5):553-67.

[44] Salthouse TA. When does age-related cognitive decline begin? Neurobiology of Aging 2009;30(4):507-14.

[45] Prinz PN, Peskind ER, Vitaliano PP, Raskind MA, Eisdorfer C, Zemcuznikov N, et al. Changes in the sleep and waking EEGs of nondemented and demented elderly subjects. Journal of the American Geriatrics Society 1982;30(2):86-93.

[46] Stewart R, Besset A, Bebbington P, Brugha T, Lindesay J, Jenkins R, et al. Insomnia comorbidity and impact and hypnotic use by age group in a national survey population aged 16 to 74 years. Sleep 2006;29(11):1391-7.

[47] Buysse DJ, Reynolds CF, Monk TH, Hoch CC. Quantification of subjective sleep quality in healthy elderly men and women using the Pittsburgh Sleep Quality Index (PSQI). Sleep: Journal of Sleep Research & Sleep Medicine 1991; 14(4):331-8.

[48] Vaz Fragoso CA, Gill TM. Sleep complaints in community-living older persons: a multifactorial geriatric syndrome. Journal of the American Geriatrics Society 2007;55(11):1853-66.

[49] Keage HAD, Banks S, Yang KL, Morgan K, Brayne C, Matthews FE. What sleep characteristics predict cognitive decline in the elderly? Sleep Medicine 2012;13(7):886-92.

[50] Mazzoni G, Gori S, Formicola G, Gneri C, Massetani R, Murri L, et al. Word recall correlates with sleep cycles in elderly subjects. Journal of Sleep Research 1999;8(3): 185-8.

[51] van der Linde R, Stephan BC, Matthews FE, Brayne C, Savva GM. Behavioural and psychological symptoms in the older population without dementia-relationship with socio-demographics, health and cognition. BMC Geriatr 2010;10:87.

[52] Bliwise DL. Sleep in normal aging and dementia. Sleep: Journal of Sleep Research & Sleep Medicine 1993;16(1):40-81.

[53] Merlino G, Piani A, Gigli GL, Cancelli I, Rinaldi A, Baroselli A, et al. Daytime sleepiness is associated with dementia and cognitive decline in older Italian adults: a population-based study. Sleep Med 2010 Apr;11(4):372-7.

[54] Bonanni L, Thomas A, Tiraboschi P, Perfetti B, Varanese S, Onofrj M. EEG comparisons in early Alzheimer's disease, dementia with Lewy bodies and Parkinson's disease with dementia patients with a 2-year follow-up. Brain 2008;131(3):690-705.

[55] Foley D, Monjan A, Masaki K, Ross W, Havlik R, White L, et al. Daytime sleepiness is associated with 3-year incident dementia and cognitive decline in older Japanese-American men. J Am Geriatr Soc 2001;49(12):1628-32.

[56] Jaussent I, Bouyer J, Ancelin ML, Berr C, Foubert-Samier A, Ritchie K, et al. Excessive sleepiness is predictive of cognitive decline in the elderly. Sleep 2012;35(9):1201-7.

[57] Petit D, Gagnon JF, Fantini ML, Ferini-Strambi L, Montplaisir J. Sleep and quantitative EEG in neurodegenerative disorders. Journal of Psychosomatic Research 2004;56(5):487-96.

[58] Loewenstein RJ, Weingartner H, Gillin JC, Kaye W, Ebert M, Mendelson WB. Disturbances of sleep and cognitive functioning in patients with dementia. Neurobiology of Aging 1983;3(4):371-7.

[59] Reynolds CF 3rd, Kupfer DJ, Taska LS, Hoch CC, Spiker DG, Sewitch DE, et al. EEG sleep in elderly depressed, demented, and healthy subjects. Biological Psychiatry 1985;20(4):431-42.

[60] Tractenberg RE, Singer CM, Kaye JA. Symptoms of sleep disturbance in persons with Alzheimer's disease and normal elderly. J Sleep Res 2005;14(2):177-85.

[61] Elwood PC, Bayer AJ, Fish M, Pickering J, Mitchell C, Gallacher JEJ. Sleep disturbance and daytime sleepiness predict vascular dementia. Journal of Epidemiology and Community Health 2011;65(9):820-4.

[62] Insana SP, Stacom EE, Montgomery-Downs HE. Actual and perceived sleep: Associations with daytime functioning among postpartum women. Physiology &Behavior 2011;102(2):234-8.

[63] Swain AM, O'Hara MW, Starr KR, Gorman LL. A prospective study of sleep, mood, and cognitive function in postpartum and nonpostpartum women. Obstetrics & Gynecology 1997;90(3):381-6.

[64] Montgomery-Downs HE, Insana SP, Clegg-Kraynok MM, Mancini LM. Normative longitudinal maternal sleep: the first 4 postpartum months. American Journal of Obstetrics and Gynecology 2010;203(5):465-81.

[65] Eidelman AI, Hoffmann NW, Kaitz M. Cognitive deficits in women after childbirth. Obstetrics and Gynecology 1993;81(5):764-7.

[66] Insana SP, Williams KB, Montgomery-Downs HE. Sleep disturbance and neurobehavioral performance among postpartum women. Sleep 2013;36(1):73-81.

[67] Greendale GA, Wight RG, Huang MH, Avis N, Gold EB, Joffe H, et al. Menopause-associated symptoms and cognitive performance: Results from the study of Women's Health Across the Nation. American Journal of Epidemiology 2010;171(11):1214-24.

[68] Kalleinen N, Polo-Kantola PA, Himanen SL, Alhola P, Joutsen A, Urrila AS, et al. Sleep and the menopause-do postmenopausal women experience worse sleep than premenopausal women? Menopause International 2008;14(3):97-104.

[69] Regestein QR, Friebely J, Shifren JL, Scharf MB, Wiita B, Carver J, et al. Self-reported sleep in postmenopausal women. Menopause 2004;11(2):198-207.

[70] Weber MT, Mapstone M, Staskiewicz J, Maki PM. Reconciling subjective memory complaints with objective memory performance in the menopausal transition. Menopause 2012;19(7):735-41.

[71] Bliwise DL. Historical change in the report of daytime fatigue. Sleep 1996;19(6):462-4.

[72] Harma M, Kandolin I. Shiftwork, age and well-being: recent developments and future perspectives. Journal of Human Ergology 2001;30(1-2):287-93.

[73] Dawson D, Reid K. Fatigue, alcohol and performance impairment. Nature 1997;388(6639):235.

[74] Poissonnet CMl, Véron M. Health effects of work schedules in healthcare professions. Journal of Clinical Nursing 2000;9(1):13-23.

[75] Spurgeon A, Harrington JM, Cooper CL. Health and safety problems associated with long working hours: a review of the current position. Occupational and Environmental Medicine 1997;54(6):367-75.

[76] Akerstedt T. Shift work and disturbed sleep/wakefulness. Occupational Medicine 2003;53(2):89-94.

[77] Bonnefond A, Harma M, Hakola T, Sallinen M, Kandolin I, Virkkala J. Interaction of age with shift-related sleep-wakefulness, sleepiness, performance, and social life. Experimental Aging Research 2006;32(2):185-208.

[78] Asaiag PE, Perotta B, Martins MdA, Tempski Pc. Quality of life, daytime sleepiness, and burnout in medical residents. Revista Brasileira de Educacao Médica 2010;34(3): 422-9.

[79] Storer JS, Floyd HH, Gill WL, Giusti CW, Ginsberg H. Effects of sleep deprivation on cognitive ability and skills of pediatrics residents. Academic Medicine 1989;64(1): 29-32.

[80] Murray D, Dodds C. The effect of sleep disruption on performance of anaesthetists-A pilot study. Anaesthesia 2003;58(6):520-5.

[81] Machi MS, Staum M, Callaway CW, Moore C, Jeong K, Suyama J, et al. The relationship between shift work, sleep, and cognition in career emergency physicians. Academic Emergency Medicine 2012;19(1):85-91.

[82] Veasey S, Rosen R, Barzansky B, Rosen I, Owens J. Sleep loss and fatigue in residency training. JAMA: The Journal of the American Medical Association 2002;288(9): 1116-24.

[83] Landrigan CP, Rothschild JM, Cronin JW, Kaushal R, Burdick E, Katz JT, et al. Effect of reducing interns' work hours on serious medical errors in intensive care units. New England Journal of Medicine 2004;351(18):1838-48.

[84] Cavallo A, Ris MD, Succop P. The night float paradigm to decrease sleep deprivation: good solution or a new problem? Ergonomics 2003;46(7):653-63.

[85] Geer RT, Jobes DR, Tew JD, Stepsis LH. Incidence of automobile accidents involving anesthesia residents after on-call duty cycles.Anesthesiology1997;87(3):A938.

[86] Lockley SW, Landrigan CP, Barger LK, Czeisler CA. When policy meets physiology: the challenge of reducing resident work hours. Clinical Orthopaedics and Related Research 2006;449:116-27.

[87] Barger LK, Ayas NT, Cade BE, Cronin JW, Rosner B, Speizer FE, et al. Impact of extended-duration shifts on medical errors, adverse events, and attentional failures. PLoS Medicine 2006;3(12):e487.

[88] Caldwell JL, Gilreath SR. Work and sleep hours of US Army aviation personnel working reverse cycle. Military Medicine 2001;166(2):159-66.

[89] Rabinowitz YG, Breitbach JE, Warner CH. Managing aviator fatigue in a deployed environment: the relationship between fatigue and neurocognitive functioning. Military Medicine 2009;174(4):358-62.

[90] Cho K. Chronic'jet lag'produces temporal lobe atrophy and spatial cognitive deficits. Nature Neuroscience 2001;4(6):567-8.

[91] Schweitzer PK, Randazzo AC, Stone K, Erman M, Walsh JK. Laboratory and field studies of naps and caffeine as practical countermeasures for sleep-wake problems associated with night work. Sleep 2006;29(1):39-50.

[92] Walsh JK, Randazzo AC, Stone KL, Schweitzer PK. Modafinil improves alertness, vigilance, and executive function during simulated night shifts. Sleep 2004 May 1;27(3):434-9.

[93] Czeisler CA, Walsh JK, Roth T, Hughes RJ, Wright KP, Kingsbury L, et al. Modafinil for excessive sleepiness associated with shift-work sleep disorder. New England Journal of Medicine 2005;353(5):476-86.

[94] Campbell SS, Dijk DJ, Boulos Z, Eastman CI, Lewy AJ, Terman M. Light treatment for sleep disorders: consensus report. III. Alerting and activating effects. J Biol Rhythms 1995 Jun;10(2):129-32.

[95] Boivin DB, James FO. Circadian adaptation to night-shift work by judicious light and darkness exposure. J Biol Rhythms 2002 Dec;17(6):556-67.

[96] Dawson D, Encel N, Lushington K. Improving adaptation to simulated night shift: timed exposure to bright light versus daytime melatonin administration. Sleep 1995 Jan;18(1):11-21.

[97] Virtanen M, Singh-Manoux A, Ferrie JE, Gimeno D, Marmot MG, Elovainio M, et al. Long working hours and cognitive function The Whitehall II Study. American Journal of Epidemiology 2009;169(5):596-605.

[98] Rouch I, Wild P, Ansiau D, Marquie JC. Shiftwork experience, age and cognitive performance. Ergonomics 2005;48(10):1282-93.

[99] Petersen RC. Mild cognitive impairment as a diagnostic entity. J Intern Med 2004 Sep;256(3):183-94.

[100] Sachdev PS, Lipnicki DM, Crawford J, Reppermund S, Kochan NA, Trollor JN, et al. Risk profiles of subtypes of mild cognitive impairment: the sydney memory and ageing study. J Am Geriatr Soc 2012 Jan;60(1):24-33.

[101] Folstein MF, Folstein SE, McHugh PR. "Mini-mental state". A practical method for grading the cognitive state of patients for the clinician. J Psychiatr Res 1975 Nov; 12(3):189-98.

[102] Potvin O, Lorrain D, Forget H, Dubé M, Grenier S, Préville M, et al. Sleep quality and 1-year incident cognitive impairment in community-dwelling older adults. Sleep 2012;35(4):491-9.

[103] Ancoli-Israel S, Ayalon L. Diagnosis and treatment of sleep disorders in older adults. Am J Geriatr Psychiatry 2006 Feb;14(2):95-103.

[104] Ancoli-Israel S, Kripke DF, Klauber MR, Mason WJ, Fell R, Kaplan O. Sleep-disordered breathing in community-dwelling elderly. Sleep 1991;14(6): 486-95.

[105] Ancoli-Israel S, Klauber MR, Butters N, Parker L. Dementia in institutionalized elderly: relation to sleep apnea. Journal of the American Geriatrics Society 1991Mar; 39(3): 258-63.

[106] Macey PM, Henderson LA, Macey KE, Alger JR, Frysinger RC, Woo MA, et al. Brain morphology associated with obstructive sleep apnea. American Journal of Respiratory and Critical Care Medicine 2002;166(10):1382-7.

[107] Kim SJ, Lee JH, Lee DY, Jhoo JH, Woo JI. Neurocognitive dysfunction associated with sleep quality and sleep apnea in patients with mild cognitive impairment. American Journal of Geriatric Psych 2011;19(4):374-81.

[108] Hoch CC, Reynolds CF 3rd, Kupfer DJ, Houck PR, Berman SR, Stack JA. Sleep-disordered breathing in normal and pathologic aging. The Journal of Clinical Psychiatry 1986;47(10):499-503.

[109] Ancoli-Israel S, Palmer BW, Cooke JR, Corey-Bloom J, Fiorentino L, Natarajan L, et al. Cognitive effects of treating obstructive sleep apnea in Alzheimer's disease: a randomized controlled study. J Am Geriatr Soc 2008 Nov;56(11):2076-81.

[110] Weaver TE, Chasens ER. Continuous positive airway pressure treatment for sleep apnea in older adults. Sleep Med Rev 2007 Apr;11(2):99-111.

[111] Vakulin A, Baulk SD, Catcheside PG, Antic NA, van den Heuvel CJ, Dorrian J, McEvoy RD. Driving simulator performance remains impaired in patients with severe OSA after CPAP treatment. J Clin Sleep Med;7(3):246-53.

[112] Boeve BF, Silber MH, Saper CB, Ferman TJ, Dickson DW, Parisi JE, et al. Pathophysiology of REM sleep behaviour disorder and relevance to neurodegenerative disease. Brain 2007;130(11):2770-88.

[113] Claassen DO, Josephs KA, Ahlskog JE, Silber MH, Tippmann-Peikert M, Boeve BF. REM sleep behavior disorder preceding other aspects of synucleinopathies by up to half a century. Neurology 2010;75(6):494-9.

[114] Schenck CH, Bundlie SR, Mahowald MW. Delayed emergence of a parkinsonian disorder in 38% of 29 older men initially diagnosed with idiopathic rapid eye movement sleep behavior disorder. Neurology 1996;46(2):388-93.

[115] Boeve BF, Silber MH, Parisi JE, Dickson DW, Ferman TJ, Benarroch EE, et al. Synucleinopathy pathology and REM sleep behavior disorder plus dementia or parkinsonism. Neurology 2003;61(1):40-5.

[116] Postuma RB, Gagnon JF, Vendette M, Fantini ML, Massicotte-Marquez J, Montplaisir J. Quantifying the risk of neurodegenerative disease in idiopathic REM sleep behavior disorder. Neurology 2009;72(15):1296-300.

[117] Postuma RB, Gagnon JF, Vendette M, Montplaisir JY. Idiopathic REM sleep behavior disorder in the transition to degenerative disease. Mov Disord 2009;24(15):2225-32.

[118] Ohayon MM, Partinen M. Insomnia and global sleep dissatisfaction in Finland. Journal of Sleep Research 2002;11(4):339-46.

[119] Diagnostic and statistical manual of mental disorders (4th Ed., text rev.). 4th ed. 2001.

[120] Ohayon MM. Epidemiology of insomnia: what we know and what we still need to learn. Sleep Medicine Reviews 2002;6(2):97-111.

[121] Fortier-Brochu E, Beaulieu-Bonneau S, Ivers H, Morin CM. Insomnia and daytime cognitive performance: a meta-analysis. Sleep Med Rev 2012 Feb;16(1):83-94.

[122] Bonnet MH, Arand DL. 24-Hour metabolic rate in insomniacs and matched normal sleepers. Sleep 1995;18(7):581-8.

[123] Crenshaw MC, Edinger JD. Slow-wave sleep and waking cognitive performance among older adults with and without insomnia complaints. Physiology &Behavior 1999;66(3):485-92.

[124] Naughton PA, Aggarwal R, Wang TT, Van Herzeele I, Keeling AN, Darzi AW, et al. Skills training after night shift work enables acquisition of endovascular technical skills on a virtual reality simulator. Journal of Vascular Surgery 2011;53(3):858-66.

[125] Leff DR, Orihuela-Espina F, Athanasiou T, Karimyan V, Elwell C, Wong J, et al. Circadian Cortical Compensation: A Longitudinal Study of Brain Function During Technical and Cognitive Skills in Acutely Sleep-Deprived Surgical Residents. Annals of Surgery 2010;252(6):1082-90.

[126] Dement W, Kleitman N. Cyclic variations in EEG during sleep and their relation to eye movements, body motility, and dreaming. Electroencephalography and Clinical Neurophysiology 1957;9(4):673-90.

[127] Karni A, Tanne D, Rubenstein BS, Askenasy JJ, Sagi D. Dependence on REM sleep of overnight improvement of a perceptual skill. Science 1994;265(5172):679-82.

[128] Spiegel R, Herzog A, Koberle S. Polygraphic sleep criteria as predictors of successful aging: an exploratory longitudinal study. Biological Psychiatry 1999;45(4):435-42.

[129] Jurado JL, Luna-Villegas G, Buela-Casal G. Normal human subjects with slow reaction times and larger time estimations after waking have diminished delta sleep. Electroencephalography and Clinical Neurophysiology 1989;73(2):124-8.

[130] Spiegel R, Koberle S, Allen SR. Significance of slow wave sleep: considerations from a clinical viewpoint. Sleep 1986;9(1):66-79.

[131] Born J, Rasch Br, Gais S. Sleep to remember. The Neuroscientist 2006;12(5):410-24.

[132] Clemens Z, Fabo D, Halasz P. Overnight verbal memory retention correlates with the number of sleep spindles. Neuroscience 2005;132(2):529-35.

[133] Van Dongen HP, Baynard MD, Maislin G, Dinges DF. Systematic interindividual differences in neurobehavioral impairment from sleep loss: evidence of trait-like differential vulnerability. Sleep 2004 May 1;27(3):423-33.

[134] Mak SK, Spurgeon P. The effects of acute sleep deprivation on performance of medical residents in a regional hospital: prospective study. Hong Kong Medical Journal 2004;10(1):14-21.

[135] Ardila A. Normal aging increases cognitive heterogeneity: Analysis of dispersion in WAIS-III scores across age. Archives of Clinical Neuropsychology 2007;22(8):1003-11.

[136] Raz N, Gunning-Dixon FM, Head D, Dupuis JH, Acker JD. Neuroanatomical correlates of cognitive aging: evidence from structural magnetic resonance imaging. Neuropsychology 1998;12(1).

[137] Gunning-Dixon FM, Raz N. The cognitive correlates of white matter abnormalities in normal aging: a quantitative review. Neuropsychology 2000;14(2):224-32.

[138] Backman L, Ginovart N, Dixon RA, Wahlin TBR, Wahlin A, Halldin C, et al. Age-related cognitive deficits mediated by changes in the striatal dopamine system. American Journal of Psychiatry 2000;157(4):635-7.

[139] The International Classification of Sleep Disorders, Fourth Edition (DSM-IV). American Academy of Sleep Medicine; European Sleep Research Society; Japanese Society of Sleep Research; Latin American Sleep Society; 1994.

[140] Horne JA, Reyner LA. Sleep related vehicle accidents. BMJ 1995 Mar 4;310(6979): 565-7.

[141] Poudel GR, Innes CR, Bones PJ, Watts R, Jones RD. Losing the struggle to stay awake: Divergent thalamic and cortical activity during microsleeps. Hum Brain Mapp 2012 Sep 24;35(1):257-69.

[142] Raichle ME, Mintun MA. Brain work and brain imaging. Annu Rev Neurosci 2006;29:449-76.

[143] Guldenmund P, Vanhaudenhuyse A, Boly M, Laureys S, Soddu A. A default mode of brain function in altered states of consciousness. Arch Ital Biol 2012 Jun;150(2-3): 107-21.

[144] Mason MF, Norton MI, Van Horn JD, Wegner DM, Grafton ST, Macrae CN. Wandering minds: the default network and stimulus-independent thought. Science 2007 Jan 19;315(5810):393-5.

[145] Raichle ME, MacLeod AM, Snyder AZ, Powers WJ, Gusnard DA, Shulman GL. A default mode of brain function. Proc Natl Acad Sci U S A 2001 Jan 16;98(2):676-82.

[146] Picchioni D, Fukunaga M, Carr WS, Braun AR, Balkin TJ, Duyn JH, et al. fMRI differences between early and late stage-1 sleep. Neurosci Lett 2008 Aug 15;441(1):81-5.

[147] Baird B, Smallwood J, Schooler JW. Back to the future: autobiographical planning and the functionality of mind-wandering. Conscious Cogn 2011 Dec;20(4):1604-11.

[148] Fox KC, Nijeboer S, Solomonova E, Domhoff GW, Christoff K. Dreaming as mind wandering: evidence from functional neuroimaging and first-person content reports. Front Hum Neurosci 2013;7:412.

[149] Dinges DF. An overview of sleepiness and accidents. Journal of Sleep Research 1995;4(s2):4-14.

[150] Mitler MM, Carskadon MA, Czeisler CA, Dement WC, Dinges DF, Graeber RC. Catastrophes, sleep, and public policy: consensus report. Sleep 1988;11(1).

[151] Ãkerstedt T, Czeisler CA, Dinges DF, Horne JA. Accidents and sleepiness: a consensus statement from the International Conference on Work Hours, Sleep and Accidents, Stockholm, 8-10 September 1994. J Sleep Res 1994;3.

[152] Arendt J, Skene DJ. Melatonin as a chronobiotic. Sleep Med Rev 2005 Feb;9(1):25-39.

[153] Luna TD. Air traffic controller shiftwork: what are the implications for aviation safety? A review. Aviation, Space, and Environmental Medicine 1997;68(1).

[154] Morris TL, Miller JC. Electrooculographic and performance indices of fatigue during simulated flight. Biological Psychology 1996;42(3):343-60.

[155] Hyman NH. Attending work hour restrictions: is it time? Archives of Surgery 2009;144(1).

[156] Pickersgill T. The European Working Time Directive for doctors in training: we will need more doctors and better organisation to comply with the law. BMJ: British Medical Journal 2001;323(7324).

[157] Ayas NT, Barger LK, Cade BE, Hashimoto DM, Rosner B, Cronin JW, et al. Extended work duration and the risk of self-reported percutaneous injuries in interns. JAMA: The Journal of the American Medical Association 2006 Sep 6;296(9):1055-62.

[158] Fletcher KE, Underwood III W, Davis SQ, Mangrulkar RS, McMahon LF Jr, Saint S. Effects of work hour reduction on residents' lives. JAMA: The Journal of the American Medical Association 2005;294(9):1088-100.

[159] Pape HC, Pfeifer R. Restricted duty hours for surgeons and impact on residents quality of life, education, and patient care: a literature review. Patient Saf Surg 2009;3(1).

[160] Reddy R, Guntupalli K, Alapat P, Surani S, Casturi L, Subramanian S. Sleepiness in medical ICU residents. Chest Journal 2009;135(1):81-5.

Chapter 2

Sleep and Cognition in Developmental Age

Marco Carotenuto and Maria Esposito

Additional information is available at the end of the chapter

http://dx.doi.org/10.5772/58967

1. Introduction

Cognitive development is the construction of thought processes, including remembering, problem solving, and decision-making, from childhood to adulthood. Moreover, it refers to how a person perceives, thinks, and gains understanding of his or her world through the interaction of genetic and learned factors. Among the areas of cognitive development are information processing, intelligence, reasoning, language development, and memory.

Historically, the cognitive development of children has been studied in a variety of ways. The oldest is through the Intelligence Quotient (IQ) based on the concept of "mental age" according to which the scores of a child of average intelligence match his or her age, while a gifted child's performance is comparable to that of an older child, and a slow learner's scores are similar to those of a younger child. IQ tests are used worldwide, but they have come under increasing criticism for defining intelligence too narrowly and for being biased with regard to race and gender.

Therefore, the study and knowledge of the various exogenous/environmental factors that could influence the cognitive development could be considered mandatory for the comprehension of the childhood general developing.

2. Sleep and cognitive processes in children

In healthy children, disturbed sleep has been associated with behavioural impairments (e.g., hyperactivity, aggression, anxiety, etc.) [1-7] and reduced neurocognitive performance (e.g., lower IQ, impaired memory, reduced academic performance, reduced attentive ability, etc.) [1,2,6,8].

Among pediatric age, growing evidence suggests the role of sleep habits as disturbing factor for influencing the cognitive development. The sleep disturbance can impact cognition as shown by the negative effects of sleep breathing disorders both in adults [9] and children [10] and as pinpointed by studies on the interaction between specific sleep stages in declarative memory functioning [11] and learning disabilities [12].

Since 1980, [13]more studies have suggested that sleep is associated with IQ levels in children, although the underlying mechanism remains still unknown. Studies involving children and adults have identified a significant relationship between poor or insufficient sleep and decreased cognitive capacity [14-26]. Furthermore, longer habitual sleep duration in healthy school-aged participants has been associated with better performance on measures of perceptual reasoning and overall IQ [23]. These findings reveal an association between sleep duration and performance on IQ tests. Actually, the DSM-5 [27] highlighted the importance of general mental abilities and of the adaptive functioning, beyond the IQ scores for the assessment of individual cognition. In this light, the social and practical domains appear to be more relevant, although the role of sleep cannot be excluded by these aspects, as showed by reports among subjects affected by intellectual disabilities (28-32).

Several Authors have proposed that sleep spindles may physiologically underpin intelligence or high-level general mental ability [33-35]. Sleep spindles are a feature of (predominantly) stage 2 Non-Rapid Eye Movement (NREM) sleep, and are characterized by recurrent and brief bursts of spindle-like EEG activity.

Moreover, spindles may be classified as either slow (10–13 Hz) or fast (13–16 Hz), with different EEG scalp topographies [36], and are both co-active also with hemodynamic responses in different cortical regions [37] and playing a strong role in the reprocessing of previously encoded information [38].Moreover, Mednick et al in 2013 have been showed as the pharmacological increase induction in spindle occurrence tend to improve memory, providing even stronger support for a mechanistic role of spindles in memory consolidation [39]. Specifically, retention of verbal informations are related to spindles recorded over frontal brain regions [40], while parietal spindles correlate with spatial memory [41].

In general, in humans the maturation of cognitive skills seems to be linked to a subsequent period of slow-wave activity (SWA), that undergoes maturation in parallel with cortical morphology [42,43] and sleep spindles (10–14 Hz) directly involved in synaptic remodeling, leading to alterations in synaptic strength and synchronized neuronal firing [44-47]

On the other hand, sleep spindle frequency in healthy school-age children seems to be negatively associated with performance on the working memory and perceptual reasoning modules of the Wechsler Intelligence Scale for Children-IV (WISC-IV) [48]. Moreover, lower sleep spindle frequency may be associated with better performance on the Intelligence perceptual reasoning and working memory WISC-IV scales, although sleep spindle amplitude, duration and density could be not directly associated with performance on the IQ test. [48]

In general in paediatric age children, sleep disturbances have been often considered as the epiphenomena of an underlying maturational disorder leading to cognitive impairments. However, cortical maturation and sleep-dependent mechanisms of brain plasticity seem to follow similar developmental trajectories, suggesting closer interactions between these two dynamic processes [42,43,49,50]. In this light, abnormal sleep activity in children might be a causal, or at least a contributing factor in cognitive and learning impairments [51,52].

Specifically, converging evidence demonstrated that sleep plays a critical role in the 'evolution' of memories [53]. In fact, once encoded, sleep-dependent memory processing can not only stabilize memories – a process classically referred to as memory consolidation – but can also enhance them and integrate them into existing memory networks, extracting key elements for retention, abstracting the gist from multi-item memories, discovering the rules governing such collections of item memories, and even modifying them in ways that facilitate the subsequent discovery of creative insights [53].

Conversely, in the declarative memory domain (i.e. the memory for facts and events, usually verbalizable and explicit), beneficial effects of post-learning sleep on performance have been highlighted using mostly verbal (word pairs) and visuospatial (e.g. memory for pictures or objects' location, virtual navigation) hippocampus-dependent learning tasks. For instance, cued recall of learned pairs of words was consistently shown better after post-learning sleep than after a similar period of time spent awake [54-61]. Additionally, sleep may help protecting recently learned memories against retroactive interference due to the acquisition of a novel and related verbal material [62,63]. Therefore, sleep would participate in memory consolidation processes more than by merely protecting novel memories from ongoing, non-specific daytime interferences and memory decay as previously advocated [64]. Likewise in the non-declarative or procedural memory domain, beneficial effects of post-learning sleep have been evidenced for the consolidation of novel skills and habits, although results are more controversial. Sleep-dependent improvements in visual discrimination skills have been consistently demonstrated using the texture discrimination task (TDT) [65-70]. Furthermore in this task, performance deteriorates over repeated practice sessions within a day reflecting the saturation of the underlying neural circuits, unless sleep is allowed between sessions [71].

In this light, performance stabilizes or even increases depending on the duration of the sleep episode and the availability of slow wave sleep (SWS) and rapid eye movement (REM) sleep [72].

A most characteristic electrophysiological feature of non-rapid eye movement (NREM) sleep is the slow oscillation, visible on scalp electroencephalography (EEG) as a biphasic wave of high amplitude and a fundamental frequency of around 1 Hz [73]. This slow oscillation is the result of the alternation of periods of extended synchronization and desynchronization of the membrane potentials of numerous cerebral cortical neurons [74].

During the hyperpolarized phase, often called "down state", neurons remain silent for up to a few hundred milliseconds. During the depolarized phase, also called "up state", neuronal spike activity takes place, often including burst firing [74]. The "up states" seem to be associated with complex and widespread neuronal network activity throughout the brain [75], including high-frequency oscillations. Especially these oscillations, and their coalescence with slow oscillations, have been implicated in network communication and systems consolidation of memory traces [76-79].

During the up states of slow oscillations, newly encoded memory representations are thought to be reactivated and redistributed, enabling a shift from temporary storage to long-term storage. Crucial for the dynamic formation of neuronal ensembles and altering of the synaptic connections during the up state is the co-occurring thalamo-cortical and cortico-cortical neuronal activity in higher frequency bands, notably the 10–15 Hz sleep spindles [80] and the >30 Hz gamma oscillations [81-83].

Over past decades, it has been evidenced that sleep can contribute to the consolidation of declarative memories in children. How and whether sleep helps in consolidating verbal and non-verbal procedural skills in this population remains a matter of debate and deserves further investigations. Dedicated studies combining comprehensive behavioural measures, neuro-physiological and/or neuroimaging recordings in healthy and pathological populations are crucially needed to unravel the mechanisms underlying the evolution of sleep-dependent memory consolidation processes during childhood. Moreover, we could speculate that neurophysiological and neuroimaging investigations may contribute to enlighten the patho-physiological associations linking abnormal sleep patterns, cognitive disturbances and impaired sleep-dependent plasticity processes throughout the developmental phase. These investigations should be conducted in parallel with the study of pathological conditions in which children present abnormal sleep patterns and cognitive deficits, such as, for a few instances, ADHD, specific language impairments and epileptic syndromes. In this framework, comparing the development of sleep-dependent plasticity markers [84] in children with or without cognitive disorders, and how this evolution interacts with cognitive functioning and/or cortical maturation, constitutes a promising field of research to understand the pathophy-siological conditions subtending the long-term disruption of cerebral plasticity processes involved in memory consolidation during sleep [84].

Moreover, the well known relationship between sleep and cognition in all ages of life suggests a key role of sleep in cognitive impairment conditions such as mental retardation [85-89], borderline intellectual functioning [32], learning [12,90], memory [91,92] and executive functions disabilities [93-95]. The approaching to the intellectual disabilities could be difficult, particularly in developmental age. In this framework sleep neuropshysiology may help the knowledge and comprehension for the functional interrelationships between the cerebral areas.

In general, the decreasing of sleep efficiency and decreased REM ratio were reported as characteristic neurophysiological signs in several developmental disabilities like Down syndrome [96,97], autism [96], Angelman syndrome [98] and in ADHD [99].

Moreover, lower sleep efficiency, higher WASO, increases in NREM sleep EEG (relative) delta and region-dependent decreases in sigma/high frequency activities were reported in subjects with Asperger syndrome [100].

Finally, reduced total sleep time, decreased sleep efficiency percentage, higher WASO, increases in frontally measured NREM sleep EEG delta power and SWS time, as well as region-dependent decreases in sigma power and reduced REM sleep percent were reported in Williams syndrome [101]. Thus, several papers are reporting similar sleep-EEG alterations in different conditions affecting intellectual functioning.

3. From childhood to adulthood: Differences and similarities in the developmental course

The differences between children and adults are legion, and how they approach and learn from new situations is clearly one of them. Purely psychological studies, ranging from the work of Piaget in the 1950s and 1960s to the ongoing work of Spelke and Carey [102], have focused on the developmental trajectory of learning capacities and the dependence of each incremental improvement on the ones preceding it. Other studies focused on the continuing development of the cerebral cortex as key to changes in learning style and intellectual development [103]. In their recent study, Wilhelm et al. suggest that at least some of the differences in how adults and children process newly acquired information result from age-dependent differences in the forms of sleep-dependent processing applied to such memories [104]. Specifically, their findings suggest that children, 8–11 years of age, show greater sleep-dependent extraction of explicit, or declarative, knowledge of the rules that govern an implicit procedural task than do adults, 18–35 years old [104].

In general, not every memory undergoes all of these forms of sleep-dependent processing, and the mechanisms that determine which ones are employed for a given memory remain poorly understood. [104].

A possible explanation of this age difference in declarative knowledge is found in the structure of children' sleep. Children not only obtained significantly more sleep than the adults (9.8 vs 6.5 hr), but spent more than twice as much of that time in deep, slow wave sleep (SWS; 39% vs 17%; 217 vs 64 min)). [105].

The suggestion that increased SWS in children might lead to better extraction or maintenance of declarative as opposed to non-declarative (e.g., procedural) knowledge has its counterpart in the suggestion found in a recent report [106] that further decreases in SWS with aging might underlie the difficulty to retain new declarative memories experienced by the elderly.

Even childhood naps may be part of this story. Among 15-month-old infants, only those who napped after a learning task retained knowledge of it the next morning [107]. Moreover, they suggested that the developmental changes in sleep architecture, with more naps, SWS, and REM sleep in children than adults, reflects parallel changes in how sleep guides the evolution of memories across the life cycle, in part enhancing explicit fact memory in children, but more abstract knowledge in adults. Perhaps sleep makes children smarter, but adults wiser [105].

The expression of slow waves undergoes remarkable changes during development, both with respect to their topographical distribution [43, 108-110], as well as with respect to their amplitude [111-113]. The amplitude of slow oscillations increases during childhood to peak shortly before puberty [112]. Conversely, a steep drop occurs during adolescence, decelerating at the age of about 17 years, after which the amplitude declines only slowly [111]. The amplitude of slow oscillations reflects the degree of synchronization by which cortical neurons switch between up and down states [88]. Although receiving much less attention, the capacity of a densely connected neuronal network to synchronize its activity may not only be reflected in the amplitude of slow oscillations, but might as well lead to more pronounced oscillations in frequency bands other than the 0.5–4 Hz range. Indeed, power in the theta (4–8 Hz) range declines across puberty and early adolescence [113]. Gaudreau et al. [114] investigated NREM sleep EEG power in a wider range of frequency bands across the age range of 6 to 60 years. They report a much higher absolute power of theta (4.0–7.75 Hz), alpha (8.0–12.0 Hz) and beta (15.25–31.0 Hz) in the group of children in the range of 6 to10 years, as compared to the groups of adolescents (range 14 to 16 years), young adults (range 19 to 29 years) and middle aged adults (range 36 to 60 years). The largest values for spindle-range power (12.25–15.0 Hz) were found in the adolescent group, suggestive of an inverted-U shape peaking somewhere between the age of about 10 years and late adolescence. Jenni and Carskadon [115] investigated developmental changes across the 0.6 to 25 Hz NREM-sleep power spectrum and found that children aged 9.6–12.9 years, as compared to children aged 11.8–15.9 years, had significantly higher absolute power not only in the low frequencies up to about 7 Hz, but also in the 12–13 Hz sigma range and 16–17 Hz low beta range. Recently, both Tarokh et al. [109, 110,116] and Baker et al. [117] applied within-subject follow-up design rather than the above-mentioned cross-sectional approaches, to confirm that changes in the sleep EEG across adolescence were not restricted to the lower frequency bands, neither to NREM sleep only. Across adolescence, the sleep EEG power decreases over a wide range of frequencies, up to the beta range for at least some derivations. In summary, the above mentioned developmental studies suggest that a wide range of cortical oscillations measured in the scalp EEG show their maximal signal to-noise ratio in late childhood, around the age of 11, where the signal of interest is the amplitude of the oscillations and the noise reflects the noise floor of scalp EEG assessment [118]. In contrast the gamma power increased on the rising slope and positive peak of the slow wave, with strongly suppression of both gamma and spindle activities during the negative peak, independently by external stiulation (i.e. acoustic) [118]

Recently, the topographic distribution of slow wave activity (SWA; EEG power between 0.75 and 4.5 Hz) during non-rapid eye movement (NREM) sleep was proposed to parallel cortical maturation from childhood through adolescence [43]. High density sleep EEG recordings in children and adolescents between 2 and 20 years of age showed that SWA exhibits a regional, age specific predominance with a developmental shift from occipital to frontal regions reaching frontal derivations only during adolescence. Strikingly, the local SWA maxima paralleled the time course of cortical gray matter [119, 120] and behavioural maturation [121] indicating that SWA may be a marker of brain maturation. This interpretation seems to be in line with the increasing number of reports showing a direct relationship between sleep slow waves and plastic cortical processes [122, 123]. More specifically, it has been hypothesized that wakefulness is associated with a significant increasing in synaptic strength, which is homeostatically rebalanced during sleep. This hypothesis was confirmed in various species examining markers of synaptic strength. A close relationship between SWA and cortical synapses has been proposed early on [124]. Although direct evidence is lacking, recent findings from animal studies or humans using current in vivo measures for cortical structure and activity support the suggestion that synaptic strength is reflected in deep sleep slow waves [125]. Several studies have shown that slow wave characteristics (SWA, topography, slope, amplitude) are closely related to maturational alterations in the cortex [42,43,49,50]. Moreover, slow waves represent synchronized activity among cortical neurons, as shown by multiunit recordings in the rat [123]. Thus, neurons show synchronized activity, the larger is the amplitude of slow waves displayed by this network. Increased synchronization is achieved by stronger synaptic connections and/or a denser network (i.e. more connections) [125].

In general it has been stated that the SWA is related to cortical plasticity [123, 126-130] (e.g., a change in strength and/or number of synapses) not only occurs because of learning processes, but also in the course of brain maturation. In fact, it was shown that SWA is not equally distributed across the scalp in children and adolescents, but exhibits local age-specific maxima [43]. Furthermore, the location of maximal SWA seems to parallel the time course of cortical maturation along the posteroanterior axis [131]. Thus, the topography of SWA may reflect cortical plasticity during development [125].

Regarding the effect of sleep deprivation, children demonstrate difficult behaviors when sleep deprived that can be stressful and impact quality of life for the entire family. Connecting sleep problems with daytime behavioral challenges may not be intuitive to parents. Adults manifest different symptoms when sleep deprived such as daytime sleepiness, psychomotor slowing and impairments in cognitive processing and memory [132]. In comparison, sleep deprivation in children is more likely to be associated with a range of emotional/behavioral disturbances, including problematic behaviors [133], attention problems [134-136], anxiety/depression [137], and hyperactivity [138, 139]. Brain maturation is a complex process [140] that begins prenatally with neural proliferation and migration and synapse formation continuing till two years of age. Myelination is an important process that begins prenatally as well but continues into adolescence with different systems myelinating at different times. The determinants of neurodevelopment and behavior rely on complex neural circuits that connect neural substrates to serve a specific function. The development of these neural circuits is still a mystery and influenced by genetic, sociocultural, medical and environmental factors [141]. The neuroanatomic substrates involved in neurobehavioral functioning span cortical, subcortical and brainstem regions and formulate complex networks which include the prefrontal cortex, amygdale and striatum. Executive functioning is highly localized to the prefrontal cortex. The amygdala is of great importance to emotional reactivity and affect and striatum to reward seeking behavior. Neuroimaging techniques reveal complex patterns of neuroanatomical functioning during specific sleep stages.

During NREM slow wave sleep, the brainstem, thalamus, basal ganglia, and prefrontal and temporal lobe regions all appear to undergo reduced activity [142]. In REM sleep, significant levels of activity are reported in the pontine tegmentum, thalamic nuclei, occipital cortex, mediobasal prefrontal lobes together with affect related regions including the amygdala, hippocampus, and anterior cingulate cortex [142]. The prefrontal cortex is relatively inactive all through sleep in contrast to its high activity during waking states [143]. This inactivity is reflected by the high voltage and slow brain wave oscillations in NREM sleep in the frontal lobes, relative to other cortical regions, suggesting that the thalamocortical input is disabled and a lower level of metabolism in the frontal lobes during NREM sleep stages is present [144]. Several investigators have suggested that sleep is particularly important for restoring pre-frontal cortical activity [145-148] however, this restorative process remains poorly understood. Neuroimaging studies showed profound effects of one night's total sleep deprivation on the blood flow to prefrontal areas which correspond to the deteriorations in daytime prefrontal task performance [149,150].

On the other hand, sleep deprivation also impacts neural circuitry underlying regulation of emotions, impulsivity and reward seeking behavior. Sleep deprived adult volunteers viewing emotional images have increased activation of the amygdala on functional neuroimaging yet weaker connection between the prefrontal cortex and the amygdala [151]. This scenario allows for uncontrolled, increased emotional response. Likewise, neurocognitive functions that involve the striatum and basal ganglia such as risk avoidance and responsiveness to rewards are also impacted by sleep deprivation. For instance, sleep deprived adults take greater risks and are less concerned about consequences of their behavior [152]. Such findings have also been noted in adolescents aged 11–13 years using functional magnetic resonance imaging (fMRI) and a guessing task with monetary rewards [153]. During reward anticipation, less activation in the caudate nucleus (part of the ventral striatum) was associated with reduced sleep time, later sleep onset time, and lower self-reported sleep quality. During reward outcome, less caudate activation was seen with later sleep onset time, earlier sleep offset time, and lower sleep quality. This findings suggested that sleep deprivation could contribute to low reactivity in reward-related brain areas in adolescents and may lead to compensatory increases in reward-driven behavior. Such findings have significant public health implications when one considers that reward seeking behaviors are associated with depressive symptoms, sensation seeking, and substance abuse in adolescents [137, 154].

4. Conclusions

The relationship between sleep and cognition is intriguing and not yet well understood.

Investigation into sleep habits in the young and the neurophysiological study of sleep (e.g. sleep macrostructure, microstructure, power spectra and CAP) may be considered as mandatory in the future for a better knowledge and comprehension of cognition development.

Author details

Marco Carotenuto* and Maria Esposito

*Address all correspondence to: marco.carotenuto@unina2.it

Sleep Clinic for Developmental Age, Department of Mental Health, Physical and Preventive Medicine, Second University of Naples, Italy

References

[1] Buckhalt, J.A., El-Sheikh, M., Keller, P.S., Kelly, R.J., 2009. Concurrent and longitudinal relations between children's sleep and cognitive functioning: the moderating role of parent education. Child Development 80, 875–892

[2] Hiscock, H., Canterford, L., Ukomunne, O.C., Wake, M., 2007. Adverse associations of sleep problems in Australian preschoolers: national population study. Pediatrics 119, 86–93.

[3] Huang, Y.S., Chen, N.H., Li, H.Y., Wu, Y.Y., Chao, C.C., Guilleminault, C., 2004. Sleep disorders in Taiwanese children with attention deficit/hyperactivity disorder. Journal of Sleep Research 13, 269–277.

[4] O'Brien, L.M., Ivanenko, A., Crabtree, V.M., Holbrook, C.R., Bruner, J.L., Klaus, C.J., Gozal, D., 2003. Sleep disturbances in children with attention deficit hyperactivity disorder. Pediatric Research 54, 237–243.

[5] Owens, J.A., Maxim, R., Nobile, C., McGuinn, M., Msall, M., 2000. Parental and self-report of sleep in children with attention-deficit/hyperactivity disorder. Archives of Pediatrics & Adolescent Medicine 154, 549–555

[6] Sadeh, A., Gruber, R., Raviv, A., 2002. Sleep, neurobehavioural functioning, and behaviour problems in school-age children. Child Development 73, 403–417

[7] Willoughby, M.T., Angold, A., Egger, H.L., 2008. Parent-reported attention-deficit/hyperactivity disorder symptomatology and sleep problems in a preschool-age pediatric clinic sample. Journal of the American Academy of Child and Adolescent Psychiatry 47, 1086–1094

[8] Randazzo, A.C., Muehlbach, M.J., Schweitzer, P.K., Walsh, J.K., 1998. Cognitive function following acute sleep restriction in children ages 10–14. Sleep 21, 861–868.

[9] Verstraeten E, Neurocognitive effects of obstructive sleep apnea syndrome, Curr. Neurol. Neurosci. Rep. 7 (2007) 161–166

[10] Kheirandish L, Gozal D, Neurocognitive dysfunction in children with sleep disorders, Dev. Sci. 9 (4) (2006) 388–399

[11] Backhaus J, Junghanns K, Born J, Hohaus K, Faasch F, Hohagen F, Impaired declarative memory consolidation during sleep in patients with primary insomnia: influence of sleep architecture and nocturnal cortisol release, Biol. Psychiatry 60 (2006) 1324–1330

[12] Bruni O, Ferri R, Novelli L, Finotti E, Terribili M, Troianiello M, Valente D,Sabatello U, Curatolo P. Slow EEG amplitude oscillations during NREM sleep and reading disabilities in children with dyslexia. Dev Neuropsychol. 2009;34(5):539-51. doi: 10.1080/87565640903133418

[13] Borrow SJ, Adam K, Chapman K, Oswald I, Hudson L, Idzikowski CJ. REM sleep and normal intelligence. Biol Psychiatry. 1980 Feb;15(1):165-9

[14] Beebe, D.W., 2011. Cognitive, behavioral, and functional consequences of inadequate sleep in children and adolescents. Pediatric Clinics of North America 58, 649–665

[15] Bell-McGinty, S., Habeck, C., Hilton, H., Rakitin, B., Scarmeas, N., Zarahn, E., et al., 2004. Identification and differential vulnerability of a neural network in sleep deprivation. Cerebral Cortex 14, 496–502

[16] Busby, K., Pivik, R.T., 1983. Sleep patterns in children of superior intelligence. Journal of Child Psychology and Psychiatry 24, 587–600

[17] Caldwell, J.A., Mu, Q., Smith, J.K., Mishory, A., Caldwell, J.L., Peters, G., et al., 2005. Are individual differences in fatigue vulnerability related to baseline differences in cortical activation? Behavioral Neuroscience 119, 694–707

[18] Chee, M.W., Choo, W.C., 2004. Functional imaging of working memory after 24 h of total sleep deprivation. The Journal of Neuroscience: The Official Journal of the Society for Neuroscience 24, 4560–4567

[19] Chee, M.W., Chuah, L.Y., Venkatraman, V., Chan, W.Y., Philip, P., Dinges, D.F., 2006. Functional imaging of working memory following normal sleep and after 24 and 35 h of sleep deprivation: correlations of fronto-parietal activation with performance. NeuroImage 31, 419–428

[20] Choo, W.C., Lee, W.W., Venkatraman, V., Sheu, F.S., Chee, M.W., 2005. Dissociation of cortical regions modulated by both working memory load and sleep deprivation and by sleep deprivation alone. NeuroImage 25, 579–587

[21] Dewald, J.F., Meijer, A.M., Oort, F.J., Kerkhof, G.A., Bogels, S.M., 2010. The influence of sleep quality, sleep duration and sleepiness on school performance in children and adolescents: a meta-analytic review. Sleep Medicine Reviews 14, 179–189

[22] Gozal, D., Kheirandish-Gozal, L., 2007. Neurocognitive and behavioral morbidity in children with sleep disorders. Current Opinion in Pulmonary Medicine 13, 505–509

[23] Gruber, R., Laviolette, R., Deluca, P., Monson, E., Cornish, K., Carrier, J., 2010. Short sleep duration is associated with poor performance on IQ measures in healthy school age children. Sleep Medicine 11, 289–294

[24] Habeck, C., Rakitin, B.C., Moeller, J., Scarmeas, N., Zarahn, E., Brown, T., et al., 2004. An event-related fMRI study of the neurobehavioral impact of sleep deprivation on performance of a delayed-match-to-sample task. Brain Research. Cognitive Brain Research 18, 306–321

[25] Voderholzer, U., Piosczyk, H., Holz, J., Landmann, N., Feige, B., Loessl, B., 2011. Sleep restriction over several days does not affect long-term recall of declarative and procedural memories in adolescents. Sleep Medicine 12, 170–178

[26] Wilhelm, I., Prehn-Kristensen, A., Born, J., 2012. Sleep-dependent memory consolidation—what can be learnt from children? Neuroscience and Biobehavioral Reviews 36, 1718–1728

[27] American Psychiatric Association: Diagnostic and Statistical Manual of Mental Disorders, Fifth Edition. Arlington, VA, American Psychiatric Association, 2013

[28] Mason TB, Arens R, Sharman J, Bintliff-Janisak B, Schultz B, Walters AS, Cater JR, Kaplan P, Pack AI. Sleep in children with Williams Syndrome. Sleep Med. 2011 Oct; 12(9):892-7. doi: 10.1016/j.sleep.2011.05.003

[29] Annaz D, Hill CM, Ashworth A, Holley S, Karmiloff-Smith A. Characterisation of sleep problems in children with Williams syndrome. Res Dev Disabil. 2011 Jan-Feb; 32(1):164-9. doi: 10.1016/j.ridd.2010.09.008

[30] Miano S, Bruni O, Aricò D, Elia M, Ferri R. Polysomnographic assessment of sleep disturbances in children with developmental disabilities and seizures. Neurol Sci. 2010 Oct;31(5):575-83. doi: 10.1007/s10072-010-0291-8

[31] Kronk R, Bishop EE, Raspa M, Bickel JO, Mandel DA, Bailey DB Jr. Prevalence, nature, and correlates of sleep problems among children with fragile X syndrome based on a large scale parent survey. Sleep. 2010 May;33(5):679-87

[32] Esposito M, Carotenuto M. Borderline intellectual functioning and sleep: the role of cyclic alternating pattern. Neurosci Lett. 2010 Nov 19;485(2):89-93. doi:10.1016/ j.neulet.2010.08.062.

[33] Bodizs, R., Kis, T. Lazar, A.S., Havran, L., Rigo, P., Clemens, Z., et al., 2005. Prediction of general mental ability based on neural oscillation measures of sleep. Journal of Sleep Research 14, 285–292

[34] Brière, M., Forest, G., Lussier, I., Godbout, G., 2000. Implicit verbal recall correlates positively with EEG sleep spindle activity. Sleep 23, A219

[35] Fogel, S.M., Nader, R., Cote, K.A., Smith, C.T., 2007. Sleep spindles and learning potential. Behavioral and Neurosciences 121, 1–10

[36] Zeitlhofer, J., Gruber, G., Anderer, P., Asenbaum, S., Schimicek, P., Saletu, B., 1997. Topographic distribution of sleep spindles in young healthy subjects. J. Sleep Res. 6 (3), 149–155

[37] Schabus, M., Dang-Vu, T.T., Albouy, G., Balteau, E., Boly, M., Carrier, J., Darsaud, A., Degueldre, C., Desseilles, M., Gais, S., et al., 2007. Hemodynamic cerebral correlates of sleep spindles during human non-rapid eye movement sleep. Proc. Natl. Acad. Sci. U. S. A. 104 (32), 13164–13169

[38] Cox R, Hofman WF, de Boer M, Talamini LM. Local sleep spindle modulations in relation to specific memory cues. NeuroImage 99 (2014) 103–110. http://dx.doi.org/ 10.1016/j.neuroimage.2014.05.028

[39] Mednick, S.C.,McDevitt, E.A.,Walsh, J.K.,Wamsley, E., Paulus, M., Kanady, J.C., Drummond, S.P., 2013. The critical role of sleep spindles in hippocampal-dependent memory: a pharmacology study. J. Neurosci. 33 (10), 4494–4504

[40] Clemens, Z., Fabó, D., Halász, P., 2005. Overnight verbal memory retention correlates with the number of sleep spindles. Neuroscience 132 (2), 529–535

[41] Clemens, Z., Fabó, D., Halász, P., 2006. Twenty-four hours retention of visuospatial memory correlates with the number of parietal sleep spindles. Neurosci. Lett. 403 (1), 52–56

[42] Buchmann, A.; Ringli, M.; Kurth, S.; Schaerer, M.; Geiger, A.; Jenni, O.G.; Huber, R. EEG sleep slow-wave activity as a mirror of cortical maturation. *Cereb. Cortex* 2011, *21*, 607–615

[43] Kurth, S.; Ringli, M.; Geiger, A.; LeBourgeois, M.; Jenni, O.G.; Huber, R. Mapping of cortical activity in the first two decades of life: A high-density sleep electroencephalogram study. *J. Neurosci.* 2010, *30*, 13211–13219

[44] Lante, F.; Toledo-Salas, J.C.; Ondrejcak, T.; Rowan, M.J.; Ulrich, D. Removal of synaptic Ca^{2+}-permeable AMPA receptors during sleep. *J. Neurosci.* 2011, *31*, 3953–3961

[45] Birtoli, B.; Ulrich, D. Firing mode-dependent synaptic plasticity in rat neocortical pyramidal neurons. *J. Neurosci.* 2004, *24*, 4935–4940

[46] Vyazovskiy, V.V.; Harris, K.D. Sleep and the single neuron: The role of global slow oscillations in individual cell rest. *Nat. Rev. Neurosci.* 2013, *14*, 443–451

[47] Kurth S, Achermann P, Rusterholz T, LeBourgeois MK. Development of Brain EEG Connectivity across Early Childhood: Does Sleep Play a Role? *Brain Sci.* 2013, *3*, 1445-1460; doi:10.3390/brainsci3041445

[48] Gruber, R., et al., The association between sleep spindles and IQ in healthy school-age children, International Journal of Psychophysiology (2013), http://dx.doi.org/10.1016/j.ijpsycho.2013.03.018

[49] Kurth, S., Jenni, O.G., Riedner, B.A., Tononi, G., Carskadon, M.A., Huber, R., 2010. Characteristics of sleep slow-waves in children and adolescents. Sleep 33, 475–480

[50] Kurth, S., Ringli, M., Lebourgeois, M.K., Geiger, A., Buchmann, A., Jenni, O.G., Huber, R., 2012. Mapping the electrophysiological marker of sleep depth reveals skill maturation in children and adolescents. NeuroImage 63, 959–965

[51] Chan, S., Baldeweg, T., Cross, J.H., 2011. A role for sleep disruption in cognitive impairment in children with epilepsy. Epilepsy & Behavior 20, 435–440

[52] Van Bogaert, P., Urbain, C., Galer, S., Ligot, N., Peigneux, P., De Tiège, X., 2011. Impact of focal interictal epileptiform discharges on behaviour and cognition in children. Neurophysiologie Clinique/Clinical Neurophysiology 42, 53–58

[53] Stickgold, R. and Walker, M.P. (2013) Sleep-dependent memory triage: evolving generalization through selective processing. Nat. Neurosci. 16, 139–145

[54] Gais, S., Born, J., 2004. Declarative memory consolidation: mechanisms acting during human sleep. Learning & Memory (Cold Spring Harbor, N.Y.) 11, 679–685

[55] Gais, S., Lucas, B., Born, J., 2006. Sleep after learning aids memory recall. Learning & Memory 13, 259–262

[56] Wilhelm, I., Diekelmann, S., Born, J., 2008. Sleep in children improves memory performance on declarative but not procedural tasks. Learning & Memory 15, 373–377

[57] Diekelmann, S., Wilhelm, I., Born, J., 2009. The whats and whens of sleep-dependent memory consolidation. Sleep Medicine Reviews 13, 309–321

[58] Diekelmann, S., Buchel, C., Born, J., Rasch, B., 2011. Labile or stable: opposing consequences for memory when reactivated during waking and sleep. Nature Neuroscience 14, 381–386

[59] Peigneux, P., Laureys, S., Fuchs, S., Destrebecqz, A., Collette, F., Delbeuck, X., Phillips, C., Aerts, J., Del Fiore, G., Degueldre, C., Luxen, A., Cleeremans, A., Maquet, P., 2003. Learned material content and acquisition level modulate cerebral reactivation during post training rapid-eye-movements sleep. NeuroImage 20, 125–134

[60] Peigneux, P., Laureys, S., Fuchs, S., Collette, F, Perrin, F., Reggers, J., Phillips, C., Degueldre, C., Del Fiore, G., Aerts, J., Luxen, A., Maquet, P., 2004 Are spatial memories strengthened in the human hippocampus during slow wave sleep? Neuron 44, 535–545

[61] Peigneux, P., Schmitz, R., Urbain, C., 2010. Sleep and forgetting. In: Della Sala, S. (Ed.), Forgetting. Psychology Press, Hove, UK

[62] Ellenbogen, J.M., Hulbert, J.C., Stickgold, R., Dinges, D.F., Thompson-Schill, S.L., 2006. Interfering with theories of sleep and memory: sleep, declarative memory, and associative interference. Current Biology 16, 1290–1294

[63] Ellenbogen, J.M., Hulbert, J.C., Jiang, Y., Stickgold, R., 2009. The sleeping brain's influence on verbal memory: boosting resistance to interference. PLoS One 4, e4117

[64] Wixted, J.T., 2004. The psychology and neuroscience of forgetting. Annual Review of Psychology 55, 235–269

[65] Gais, S., Plihal, W., Wagner, U., Born, J., 2000. Early sleep triggers memory for early visual discrimination skills. Nature Neuroscience 3, 1335-1139

[66] Gais, S., Rasch, B., Wagner, U., Born, J., 2008. Visual-procedural memory consolidation during sleep blocked by glutamatergic receptor antagonists. Journal of Neuroscience 28, 5513–5518

[67] Karni, A., Tanne, D., Rubenstein, S., Askenasy, J.J.M., Sagi, D., 1994. Dependence on REM sleep of overnight improvement of a perceptual skill. Science 265, 679–682

[68] Karni, A., Meyer, G., Rey-Hipolito, C., Jezzard, P., Adams, M.M., Turner, R., Ungerleider, L.G., 1998. The acquisition of skilled motor performance: fast and slow experience-driven changes in primary motor cortex. Proceedings of the National Academy of Sciences of the United States of America 95, 861–868

[69] Stickgold, R., 2005. Sleep-dependent memory consolidation. Nature 437, 1272–1278

[70] Stickgold, R., Whidbee, D., Schirmer, B., Patel, V., Hobson, J.A., 2000. Visual discrimination task improvement: a multi-step process occurring during sleep. Journal of Cognitive Neuroscience 12, 246–254

[71] Mednick, S.C., Nakayama, K., Cantero, J.L., Atienza, M., Levin, A.A., Pathak, N., Stickgold, R., 2002. The restorative effect of naps on perceptual deterioration. Nature Neuroscience 5, 677–681

[72] Mednick, S.C., Nakayama, K., Stickgold, R., 2003. Sleep-dependent learning: a nap is as good as a night. Nature Neuroscience 6, 697–698

[73] Achermann, P., Borbély, A.A., 1997. Low-frequency (b1 Hz) oscillations in the human sleep electroencephalogram. Neuroscience 81, 213–222

[74] Steriade, M., Nuñez, A., Amzica, F., 1993. A novel slow (b1 Hz) oscillation of neocortical neurons in vivo: depolarizing and hyperpolarizing components. Journal of Neuroscience 13, 3252–3265

[75] Volgushev, M., Chauvette, S, Timofeev, I., 2011. Long-range correlation of the membrane potential in neocortical neurons during slow oscillation. Progress in Brain Research 193, 181–199

[76] Diekelmann, S., Born, J., 2010. The memory function of sleep. Nature Reviews. Neuroscience 11, 114–126

[77] Mölle, M., Born, J., 2011. Slow oscillations orchestrating fast oscillations and memory consolidation. Progress in Brain Research 193, 93–110

[78] Schwindel, C.D., McNaughton, B.L., 2011. Hippocampal–cortical interactions and the dynamics of memory trace reactivation. Progress in Brain Research 193, 163–177

[79] Van Someren, E.J.W., Van Der Werf, Y.D., Roelfsema, P.R., Mansvelder, H.D., Lopes da Silva, F.H., Da Silva, F.H.L., 2011. Slow brain oscillations of sleep, resting state, and vigilance. Progress in Brain Research 193, 3–15

[80] Rosanova, M., Ulrich, D., 2005. Pattern-specific associative long-term potentiation induced by a sleep spindle-related spike train. Journal of Neuroscience 25, 9398–9405

[81] Steriade, M., Amzica, F., Contreras, D., 1996. Synchronization of fast (30–40 Hz) spontaneous cortical rhythms during brain activation. Journal of Neuroscience 16, 392–417

[82] Mena-Segovia, J., Bolam, J.P., 2011. Phasic modulation of cortical high-frequency oscillations by pedunculopontine neurons. Progress in Brain Research 193, 85–92

[83] Mena-Segovia, J., Sims, H.M., Magill, P.J., Bolam, J.P., 2008. Cholinergic brainstem neurons modulate cortical gamma activity during slow oscillations. Journal of Physiology (London) 586, 2947–2960

[84] Urbain, C., et al., Pathophysiology of sleep-dependent memory consolidation processes in children, International Journal of Psychophysiology (2013), http://dx.doi.org/10.1016/j.ijpsycho.2013.06.022

[85] Stores G, Stores R. Sleep disorders and their clinical significance in children with Down syndrome. Dev Med Child Neurol. 2013 Feb;55(2):126-30. doi:10.1111/j.1469-8749.2012.04422.x.

[86] Anders T, Iosif AM, Schwichtenberg AJ, Tang K, Goodlin-Jones B. Sleep and daytime functioning: a short-term longitudinal study of three preschool-age comparison groups. Am J Intellect Dev Disabil. 2012 Jul;117(4):275-90. doi: 10.1352/1944-7558-117.4.275.

[87] Miamoto CB, Pereira LJ, Ramos-Jorge ML, Marques LS. Prevalence and predictive factors of sleep bruxism in children with and without cognitive impairment. Braz Oral Res. 2011 Sep-Oct;25(5):439-45

[88] Ringli M, Huber R. Developmental aspects of sleep slow waves: linking sleep, brain maturation and behavior. Prog Brain Res. 2011;193:63-82. doi:10.1016/B978-0-444-53839-0.00005-3

[89] Buckley AW, Rodriguez AJ, Jennison K, Buckley J, Thurm A, Sato S, Swedo S. Rapid eye movement sleep percentage in children with autism compared with children with developmental delay and typical development. Arch Pediatr Adolesc Med. 2010 Nov;164(11):1032-7. doi: 10.1001/archpediatrics.2010.202

[90] Mercier L, Pivik RT, Busby K. Sleep patterns in reading disabled children. Sleep. 1993 Apr;16(3):207-15.

[91] Dijk DJ. Sleep in children, sleep spindles, and the metrics of memory. J Sleep Res. 2013 Apr;22(2):119-20. doi: 10.1111/jsr.12052

[92] Kopasz M, Loessl B, Hornyak M, Riemann D, Nissen C, Piosczyk H, Voderholzer U. Sleep and memory in healthy children and adolescents-a critical review. Sleep Med Rev. 2010 Jun;14(3):167-77. doi: 10.1016/j.smrv.2009.10.006

[93] Bernier A, Beauchamp MH, Bouvette-Turcot AA, Carlson SM, Carrier J. Sleep and Cognition in Preschool Years: Specific Links to Executive Functioning. Child Dev. 2013 Feb 24. doi: 10.1111/cdev.12063

[94] Hahn C, Cowell JM, Wiprzycka UJ, Goldstein D, Ralph M, Hasher L, Zelazo PD. Circadian rhythms in executive function during the transition to adolescence: the effect of synchrony between chronotype and time of day. Dev Sci. 2012 May;15(3):408-16. doi: 10.1111/j.1467-7687.2012.01137.x

[95] Barnes ME, Gozal D, Molfese DL. Attention in children with obstructive sleep apnoea: an event-related potentials study. Sleep Med. 2012 Apr;13(4):368-77. doi: 10.1016/j.sleep.2011.06.007

[96] Diomedi M, Curatolo P, Scalise A, Placidi F, Caretto F, Gigli GL. (1999) Sleep abnormalities in mentally retarded autistic subjects: Down's syndrome with mental retardation and normal subjects. Brain Dev. 21(8):548-53

[97] Miano S, Bruni O, Elia M, Scifo L, Smerieri A, Trovato A, et al. (2008) Sleep phenotypes of intellectual disability: a polysomnographic evaluation in subjects with Down syndrome and Fragile-X syndrome. Clin Neurophysiol.;119(6):1242-7

[98] Miano S, Bruni O, Leuzzi V, Elia M, Verrillo E, Ferri R. (2004) Sleep polygraphy in Angelman syndrome. Clin Neurophysiol. 115(4):938-45

[99] Sobanski E, Schredl M, Kettler N, Alm B. (2008) Sleep in adults with attention deficit hyperactivity disorder (ADHD) before and during treatment with methylphenidate: a controlled polysomnographic study. Sleep. 31(3):375-81

[100] Lazar AS, Lazar ZI, Biro A, Gyori M, Tarnok Z, Prekop C, Keszei A, Stefanik K, Gadoros J, Halasz P, Bodizs R. (2010) Reduced fronto-cortical brain connectivity during NREM sleep in Asperger syndrome: an EEG spectral and phase coherence study. Clin Neurophysiol. 121(11):1844-54

[101] Gombos F, Bodizs R, Kovacs I. (2011) Atypical sleep architecture and altered EEG spectra in Williams syndrome. J Intellect Disabil Res;55(3):255-62

[102] Spaepen, E. et al. (2011) Number without a language model. Proc. Natl. Acad. Sci. U.S.A. 108, 3163–3168

[103] Shaw, P. et al. (2006) Intellectual ability and cortical development in children and adolescents. Nature 440, 676–679

[104] Wilhelm, I. et al. (2013) The sleeping child outplays the adult's capacity to convert implicit into explicit knowledge. Nat. Neurosci. 16, 391–393

[105] Stickgold R. Early to bed: how sleep benefits children's memory. Trends Cogn Sci. 2013 Jun;17(6):261-2. doi: 10.1016/j.tics.2013.04.006

[106] Mander, B.A. et al. (2013) Prefrontal atrophy, disrupted NREM slow waves and impaired hippocampal-dependent memory in aging. Nat. Neurosci. 16, 357–364

[107] Hupbach, A. et al. (2009) Nap-dependent learning in infants. Dev. Sci. 12, 1007–1012

[108] Jenni, O.G., Van Reen, E., Carskadon, M.A., 2005. Regional differences of the sleep electroencephalogram in adolescents. Journal of Sleep Research 14, 141–147

[109] Tarokh, L., Carskadon, M.A., 2010. Developmental changes in the human sleep EEG during early adolescence. Sleep 33, 801–809

[110] Tarokh, L., Carskadon, M.A., Achermann, P., 2010. Developmental changes in brain connectivity assessed using the sleep EEG. Neuroscience 171, 622–634

[111] Feinberg, I., Campbell, I.G., 2010. Sleep EEG changes during adolescence: an index of a fundamental brain reorganization. Brain and Cognition 72, 56–65

[112] Feinberg, I., Thode, H.C., Chugani, H.T., March, J.D., 1990. Gamma distribution model describes maturational curves for delta wave amplitude, cortical metabolic rate and synaptic density. Journal of Theoretical Biology 142, 149–161

[113] Feinberg, I., De Bie, E., Davis, N.M., Campbell, I.G., 2011. Topographic differences in the adolescent maturation of the slow wave EEG during NREM sleep. Sleep 34, 325–333

[114] Gaudreau, H., Carrier, J., Montplaisir, J., 2001. Age-related modifications of NREM sleep EEG: from childhood to middle age. Journal of Sleep Research 10, 165–172

[115] Jenni, O.G., Carskadon, M.A., 2004. Spectral analysis of the sleep electroencephalogram during adolescence. Sleep 27, 774–783

[116] Tarokh, L., Reen, E. Van, Lebourgeois, M., Seifer, R., Carskadon, M.A., Van Reen, E., 2011. Sleep EEG provides evidence that cortical changes persist into late adolescence. Sleep 34, 1385–139

[117] Baker, F.C., Turlington, S.R., Colrain, I., 2012. Developmental changes in the sleep electroencephalogram of adolescent boys and girls. Journal of Sleep Research 21, 59–67

[118] Piantoni, G., et al., Modulation of gamma and spindle-range power by slow oscillations in scalp sleep EEG of children, International Journal of Psychophysiology (2013), http://dx.doi.org/10.1016/j.ijpsycho.2013.01.017

[119] Gogtay, N., Giedd, J.N., Lusk, L., Hayashi, K.M., Greenstein, D., Vaituzis, A.C., Nugent, T.F., Herman, D.H., Clasen, L.S., Toga, A.W., Rapoport, J.L., Thompson, P.M., 2004. Dynamic mapping of human cortical development during childhood through early adulthood. Proceedings of the National Academy of Sciences of the United States of America 101, 8174–8179

[120] Sowell, E.R., Thompson, P.M., Leonard, C.M., Welcome, S.E., Kan, E., Toga, A.W., 2004. Longitudinal mapping of cortical thickness and brain growth in normal children. Journal of Neuroscience 24, 8223–8231

[121] Luna, B., Sweeney, J.A., 2004. The emergence of collaborative brain function: FMRI studies of the development of response inhibition. Annals of the New York Academy of Sciences 1021, 296–309

[122] Tononi, G., Cirelli, C., 2006. Sleep function and synaptic homeostasis. Sleep Medicine Reviews 10, 49–62

[123] Vyazovskiy, V.V., Olcese, U., Lazimy, Y.M., Faraguna, U., Esser, S.K., Williams, J.C., Cirelli, C., Tononi, G., 2009. Cortical firing and sleep homeostasis. Neuron 63, 865–878

[124] Feinberg, I., 1982. Schizophrenia: caused by a fault in programmed synaptic elimination during adolescence? Journal of Psychiatric Research 17, 319–334

[125] Ringli, M., et al., The sleep EEG topography in children and adolescents shows sex differences in language areas, International Journal of Psychophysiology (2013), http://dx.doi.org/10.1016/j.ijpsycho.2013.04.008

[126] Huber, R.,Graf, T., Cote, K.A.,Wittmann, L., Gallmann, E.,Matter, D., Schuderer, J., Kuster,N., Borbely, A.A., Achermann, P., 2000. Exposure to pulsed high-frequency electromagnetic field during waking affects human sleep EEG. NeuroReport 11, 3321–3325

[127] Huber, R., Ghilardi, M.F., Massimini, M., Tononi, G., 2004. Local sleep and learning. Nature 430, 78–81

[128] Huber, R., Ghilardi, M.F., Massimini, M., Ferrarelli, F., Riedner, B.A., Peterson, M.J., Tononi, G., 2006. Arm immobilization causes cortical plastic changes and locally decreases sleep slow wave activity. Nature Neuroscience 9, 1169–1176

[129] Huber, R., Mäki, H., Rosanova, M., Casarotto, S., Canali, P., Tononi, G., Massimini, M., 2013. Human cortical excitability increases with time awake. Cerebral Cortex 23, 332–338

[130] Vyazovskiy, V.V., Cirelli, C., Pfister-Genskow, M., Faraguna, U., Tononi, G., 2008. Molecular and electrophysiological evidence for net synaptic potentiation in wake and depression in sleep. Nature Neuroscience 11, 200–208

[131] Shaw, P., Kabani, N.J., Lerch, J.P., Eckstrand, K., Lenroot, R., Gogtay, N., Greenstein, D., Clasen, L., Evans, A., Rapoport, J.L., Giedd, J.N., Wise, S.P., 2008. Neurodevelopmental trajectories of the human cerebral cortex. Journal of Neuroscience 28, 3586–3594

[132] O'Brien, L.M., Holbrook, C.R.,Mervis, C.B., Klaus, C.J., Bruner, J.L., Raffield, T.J., Rutherford, J., Mehl, R.C., Wang,M., Tuell, A., Hume, B.C., Gozal, D., 2003. Sleep and neurobehavioral characteristics of 5-to 7-year-old children with parentally reported symptoms of attention-deficit/hyperactivity disorder. Pediatrics 111, 554–563

[133] Aronen, E.T., Paavonen, E.J., Fjallberg, M., Soininen, M., Torronen, J., 2000. Sleep and psychiatric symptoms in school-age children. Journal of the American Academy of Child and Adolescent Psychiatry 39, 502–508

[134] Fallone, G., Acebo, C., Seifer, R., Carskadon, M.A., 2005. Experimental restriction of sleep opportunity in children: effects on teacher ratings. Sleep 28, 1561–1567

[135] Sadeh, A., Gruber, R., Raviv, A., 2003. The effects of sleep restriction and extension on schoolage children: what a difference an hour makes. Child Development 74, 444–455

[136] Sadeh, A., Pergamin, L., Bar-Haim, Y., 2006. Sleep in children with attention-deficit hyperactivity disorder: ameta-analysis of polysomnographic studies. Sleep Medicine Reviews 10, 381–398

[137] Forbes, E.E., Bertocci, M.A., Gregory, A.M., Ryan, N.D., Axelson, D.A., Birmaher, B., Dahl, R.E., 2008. Objective sleep in pediatric anxiety disorders and major depressive disorder. 47, 148–155

[138] Touchette, E., Petit, D., Seguin, J.R., Boivin, M., Tremblay, R.E., Montplaisir, J.Y., 2007. Associations between sleep duration patterns and behavioral/cognitive functioning at school entry. Sleep 30, 1213–1219

[139] Touchette, E., Cote, S.M., Petit, D., Liu, X., Boivin, M., Falissard, B., Tremblay, R.E., Montplaisir, J.Y., 2009. Short nighttime sleep-duration and hyperactivity trajectories in early childhood. Pediatrics 124, e985–993

[140] Giedd, J., 1999. Brain development, IX: human brain growth. The American Journal of Psychiatry 156, 4

[141] Rice, D., Barone Jr., S., 2000. Critical periods of vulnerability for the developing nervous system: evidence from humans and animal models. Environmental Health Perspectives 108 (Suppl. 3), 511–533

[142] Nofzinger, E.A., 2005. Functional neuroimaging of sleep. Seminars in Neurology 25, 9–18

[143] Binder, J.R., Frost, J.A., Hammeke, T.A., Bellgowan, P.S., Rao, S.M., Cox, R.W., 1999. Conceptual processing during the conscious resting state. A functional MRI study. Journal of Cognitive Neuroscience 11, 80–95

[144] Maquet, P., Degueldre, C., Delfiore, G., Aerts, J., Peters, J.M., Luxen, A., Franck, G., 1997. Functional neuroanatomy of human slow wave sleep. Journal of Neuroscience 17, 2807–2812

[145] Dahl, R.E., 1996. The impact of inadequate sleep on children's daytime cognitive function. Seminars in Pediatric Neurology 3, 44–50

[146] Dahl, R.E., 1996. The regulation of sleep and arousal: development and psychopathology. Development and Psychopathology 8, 3–27

[147] Horne, J.A., 1993. Human sleep, sleep loss and behaviour. Implications for the prefrontal cortex and psychiatric disorder. The British Journal of Psychiatry 162, 413–419

[148] Muzur, A., Pace-Schott, E.F., Hobson, J.A., 2002. The prefrontal cortex in sleep. Trends in Cognitive Science 6, 475–481

[149] Drummond, S.P., Brown, G.G., Stricker, J.L., Buxton, R.B.,Wong, E.C., Gillin, J.C., 1999. Sleep deprivation-induced reduction in cortical functional response to serial subtraction. Neuroreport 10, 3745–3748

[150] Thomas, M., Sing, H., Belenky, G., Holcomb, H., Mayberg, H., Dannals, R., Wagner, H., Thorne, D., Popp, K., Rowland, L., Welsh, A., Balwinski, S., Redmond, D., 2000. Neural basis of alertness and cognitive performance impairments during sleepiness. I. Effects of 24 h of sleep deprivation on waking human regional brain activity. Journal of Sleep Research 9, 335–352

[151] van der Helm, E., Gujar, N., Walker, M.P., 2010. Sleep deprivation impairs the accurate recognition of human emotions. Sleep 33, 335–342

[152] Dijk, D.J., 2011. Risk-taking and other effects of sleep loss on brain function and behaviour. Journal of Sleep Research 20, 375–376

[153] Holm, S.M., Forbes, E.E., Ryan, N.D., Phillips, M.L., Tarr, J.A., Dahl, R.E., 2009. Reward related brain function and sleep in pre/early pubertal and mid/late pubertal adolescents. The Journal of Adolescent Health 45, 326–334

[154] Nelson, E.E., Leibenluft, E., McClure, E.B., Pine, D.S., 2005. The social re-orientation of adolescence: a neuroscience perspective on the process and its relation to psychopathology. Psychological Medicine 35, 163–174

Section 2

Parasomnias - Sleep-Related Sexual Behaviour

Chapter 3

An Essay on Sleep-Related Sexual Behaviours and Offences Related to Sexual Behaviours

Chris Idzikowski

Additional information is available at the end of the chapter

http://dx.doi.org/10.5772/59140

1. Introduction

The aim of this chapter is to consider mainly the deep sleep parasomnias associated with sexual behaviour (known variously as sexsomnia, sleep sex, etc, see below) that may lead to non-consensual behaviour resulting in criminal charges.

Most jurisdictions will acquit a defendant if a court accepts that the criminal behaviour occurred whilst they were asleep-that is they were 'sleepwalking' or in a 'somnambulistic' state. It is said that Hippocrates and Aristotle were aware of the condition; that Galen wrote in *De motu musculorum* "that he once spent a whole night walking about in his sleep, awakening only after he struck a stone in his way" and that the philosopher Diogenes Laërtius "was said to read, to write, and to correct his works while asleep" [1], similar to one of John Polidori's cases [2]. Umanath et al also note that Polish intellectual Joannes Jonstonus in his 1632 *Thaumatographia naturalis* had a section on "Of Walkers in the Night" [1]. In England King James II in the seventeenth century pardoned Colonel Cheyney Culpeper for shooting a guardsman and his horse with a blunderbuss [1, 3]. (It should be noted that blunderbusses are not very accurate though very effective at short range.)

Sexual relations are complex across a range of dimensions [4] which could impact on reporting of sexual crimes, both historically and now. Some may be clouded in confusion-as for example, with the 'Old Hag' (an *incubus*?) in sleep paralysis (when the muscles of the body are temporarily paralysed around the time of awakening) [5]. Schenck et al do cover sleep paralysis mainly in the context of narcolepsy though [6]. In their appendix they had to resort to quoting Tess's experience in Thomas Hardy's *Tess of the d'Urbervilles* (1891) [7] to provide some historical though literature-based context.

Putting forward a sleep-related sexual behaviour (SRSB) as a defence is relatively new and has emerged within the last two decades. Whilst the literature shows Bowden [8] reacting to Buchanan's report of a case of somnambulistic indecent exposure [9] by pointing out that Motet in an 1897 article in the *Annales d'Hygiène et de Médecine Légale* described a similar case, this is not the type of sexual offence considered in this chapter (the advice generally being wear pyjamas or nighties if you are a sleepwalker). As a side note, Motet's case was interesting as the court acquitted the defendant on the basis that a somnambulistic state was confirmed by hypnotism. Using the England and Wales Sexual Offences Act 2003 as a guide the type of offences considered are rape, sexual assault by penetration, sexual assault, *etc*, those offences where consent is as much of an issue as the behaviour. Both Shapiro (Canada) [10, 11] and Guilleminault (U.S.) [12] were the first to describe case series of SRSBs (though there had previously been sporadic case reports, e.g. Wong: masturbation [13] and forensic cases, e.g. Fenwick [14]), which eventually led to both Schenck et al's 2007 comprehensive, thorough and critical review of the whole area [6].

Legal procedures have evolved to deal with sleep-related violent behaviour but SRSB has only recently been described so existing laws have to be applied to these cases. Given that courts have no experience with these cases inevitably means that expert guidance is needed. There are, however, as this essay flags problems, e.g.1) laws are inconsistent with respect to sleep-related violence and 2) sleep research is in its infancy and has difficulty answering the questions that courts may pose. To examine these problems the recently published 2014 3rd edition of the International Classification of Sleep Disorders [15] will be used as a springboard to explore SRSB. This is followed by an examination of existing SRSB literature, and the professional guidelines that have evolved to manage these cases. The problem of matching the different possible medical (mainly psychiatric) models of these disorders with the different legal models of a defendant [16] and the lack of an ontological basis with which to link these two professional domains will be deferred to another essay.

2. The international classification of sleep disorders 3rd edition [2014] [15]

The International Classification of Sleep Disorders Diagnostic and Coding Manual, 3rd edition [2014] (ICSD3) [15] lists more than 60 different sleep disorders. This is a reduction to the number of disorders listed in the previous manual, published 2007, which had 80 but more than the original manual published 1990. The reduction reflects refinements in the classification and pooling some categories which were better covered by umbrella terms.

The sleep disorders are roughly classified into insomnias (inability to sleep), hypersomnias (inability to remain awake), sleep-related breathing disorders (SRBs) and the parasomnias (unwanted or abnormal behaviours during sleep) see Table 1. The parasomnias are the main group of interest in ICSD3 [17]. There are overlaps (e.g. treatment of SRBs may trigger the (re-) emergence of a parasomnia [18] or SRBs may mimic parasomnias [19], or hypersomnias like narcolepsy [20, 21].

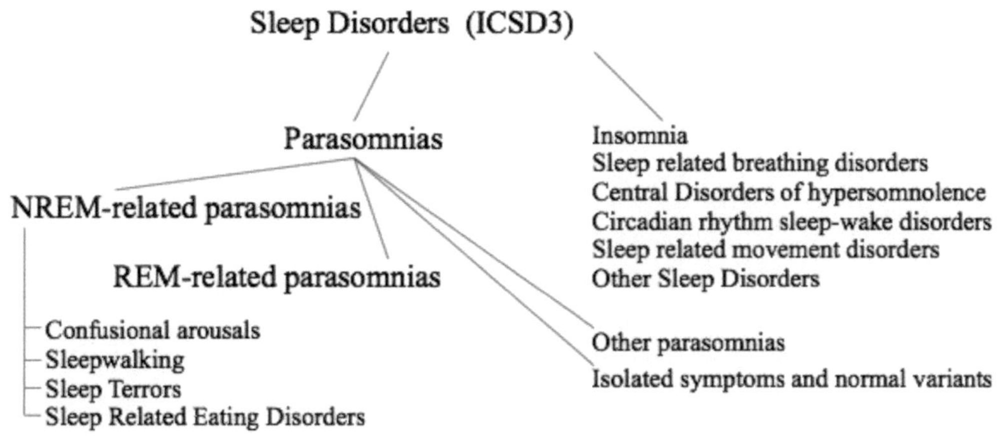

Figure 1. Sleep Disorders (ICSD3)

The parasomnias are further divided into REM (Rapid Eye Movement) and NREM (Non-REM) – Figure 1; and again there are overlaps such as Parasomnia Overlap Disorder. The NREM Disorders of Arousal include Confusional Arousals, Sleepwalking and Night Terrors. These disorders all have similar characteristics and are distinguished thus: **Confusional arousals** are characterised by mental confusion or confused behaviour that occurs while the person is in bed and there is an absence of terror or ambulation outside of the bed. **Sleepwalking** is associated with ambulation and other behaviours out of bed whilst **Sleep (Night) Terrors** are characterised "by episodes of abrupt terror, typically beginning with an alarming vocalization such as a frightening scream" and "There is intense fear and signs of autonomic arousal, including mydriasis, tachycardia, tachypnea, and diaphoresis during an episode.

Disorders of Arousal (From NREM Sleep) - confusional arousals, sleepwalking, sleep terrors (including SRSBs)	
share similar	
1	genetic and familial patterns
2	pathophysiology of partial arousals from deep sleep
3	priming by sleep deprivation and bio-psychosocial stressors
and are	
1	not secondary to psychiatric disorders
2	not generally secondary to neuropathology or head injury
3	associated with absent or minimal cognitive functioning
4	associated with amnesia for the prior episode
5	may be triggered by sound, touch, or other stimuli

Table 1. Disorders of Arousal (From NREM Sleep) — Confusional arousals, sleepwalking, sleep terrors (including SRSBs) share similar:

As with many diagnostic schemes the frequency of a sign or symptom leads to a classification rule. The problem in many legal cases is that all the signs and symptoms for a recognised (medical) mental disorder may be present but a single instance is insufficient to warrant a 'diagnosis'.

3. Disorders of arousal

Disorders of arousal lead to behaviours that are usually initiated during partial arousals from (deep) slow wave (N3) sleep. "Most episodes are brief, but they may last as long as 30 to 40 minutes [in some children]." ICSD3 notes that most sleepwalking occurs in *children*. "They are especially prevalent among children and adults younger than 35 years." Also: "The prevalence of confusional arousals in children three to 13 years of age in a large population-based study was 17.3%. Lifetime prevalence of confusional arousals has recently been reported as 18.5% (16.1-20.9 confidence interval). The prevalence among adults older than 15 years is 2.9% to 4.2%".

The behaviours can be simple or complex, well-learned or automated or instinctive behaviour of which the person is thought to be unaware and usually is completely amnesic; there is either no, or relatively sparse mental content. Actions are not necessarily completed. Awakening is difficult and slow-this effect is known as sleep inertia (and has been called sleep drunkeness). "Sleep talking and shouting may accompany these events. The eyes are usually open during an episode and, not uncommonly, are wide open with a confused "glassy" stare." Someone with "a disorder of arousal may be very difficult to awaken and, when awakened, is often confused. There is usually amnesia for these episodes, although adults may remember fragments of episodes. Dream-like mentation is sometimes reported in adults. Other high-level cognitive functions such as attention, planning, social interaction, and intent are absent."

Sleepwalking tends to run in families. A twin study looking at how genetic and environmental factors affect sleepwalking looked at 11, 220 subjects including 1, 045 monozygotic (genetically identical) twins and 1, 899 dizygotic (50% of gene factors shared) twins. Childhood sleep-walking was more frequent in women 9% saying they experienced it "sometimes" or "often" compared to 8%" of men. Childhood sleepwalkers can continue walking as adults. 24.6% of men and for 18.3% of women continued to walk if they had walked frequently as children [22]. Of adult men sleepwalkers 88.9% had a positive history of sleepwalking in childhood, and in women, 84.5%. For both men and women those who never walked in their sleep as children did so rarely has adults-0.6%.In a separate study, immediate relatives of sleepwalkers were shown to have at least a 10-fold increased likelihood of sleepwalking over that of the general population. There are no studies on genetic similarity. The highest correlations in both children and adults between parasomnias were between sleep talking with sleepwalking, nightmares, and bruxism (tooth grinding) [22].

It is not clear why sleepwalking should decline during adolescence. Certainly children have much more deep sleep than adults and the duration of deep sleep declines during adolescence.

http://dx.doi.org/10.5772/59140

What triggers sleepwalking is also an area of debate. During deep sleep the thalamus which is the main sensory relay in the brain goes into an idling or neutral state so less sensory information is passed up to the cortex. The cortex reacts to stimuli so with less stimuli the less there is to respond to. As the areas of brain that handle automatic or well-learned behaviour have not shut down but are also in a neutral state, the person just continues to sleep. However, if there is an interruption of breathing or some other stimulus then the learned behaviour may be triggered. As the rational part of the brain is switched off there is nothing to prevent the behaviour, the walk, beginning. Recent research on adult sleepwalkers showed that sleepwalkers thought that stressful events during the day triggered sleepwalking 52% of the time. Other important triggers that were reported were: strong positive emotions 42%, prior sleep deprivation 27%, alcohol 12% and intense physical activity 5% [23]. However, it has been suggested recall bias may have affected these results [24].

Zadra has highlighted some misconceptions concerning somnambulism that have arisen over time: 1) that it has no daytime consequences; apparently there are, patients are more somnolent and have daytime functioning anomalies, 2) somnambulism is characterised by episodic amnesia-this appears not to be the case and 3) somnambulism is an automatic behaviour arising in the absence of dreamlike mental activity-again untrue, it has always been known that dream mentation is not exclusively related to REM sleep and Montplaisir's group has noted mentation in somnambulists [25]. These ambiguities lead to disagreements in classification and diagnostic committees. For legal cases this is a problem as factors that are considered as significant may in fact not be. There is also a problem with working clinician's experience, particularly those who are not engaged at sleep centres and even those have the difficulty of not actually knowing what patients do in their homes as patients, on the whole, do not have the capacity to walk in sleep centres.

3.1. Sleep-related violence

NREM Disorders of arousal are not inevitably associated with (criminally) violent behaviour. In a cohort of 64 of his patients Moldofsky noted with 89% sensitivity, 80% specificity and 81% diagnostic accuracy violence was associated with being male and having less than 2% stage 4 sleep (similar to N3, refer to table 4) [26]. Also associated was experiencing more stressors, drinking excessive caffeinated beverages and abusing drugs. A UK population study on 2, 078 men and 2, 894 women reported 1997 noted a frequency of 2% [27]. A larger sample of 19, 961 participants was polled 2010 in Finland, Germany, Italy, Portugal, Spain and the UK and found the frequency was 1.7% of the population [28]. The perpetrators were younger than 35. 61.5% noted vivid dreams during the episodes, though the highest frequency was observed with subjects suffering from sleepwalking and sleep terrors. It is notable that only 12.3% of these subjects reported their problems to a physician. Guilleminault reviewed his violent cases in 1998 comprising of 48 patients with REM Behaviour Disorder (who will not be discussed in this essay), 44 young somnambulistic patients (mean age 18+/-5 years) and 27 older subjects [29]. His review is preceded with pertinent questions for the forensic area:"*Is the subject ever 'asleep' during violent acts, do the events occur out of sleep, or is there an intermediate or borderland period between sleep and wake? At what point does full alertness occur? Is there a decrease or absence of judgment when violent actions occur within this ill-defined borderland between wake and sleep? Based on available data, if one accepts the existence of this borderland of sleep and abnormal states of alertness, how long could this "abnormal state" last? Is there some event during sleep that influences the violent behavior? Is the state of alertness during the abnormal behavior different from "normal" wake, and, if different, how and based on what objective information?"* Perhaps the review not surprisingly could not answer the questions but characterise many of the behaviours that can occur and further noted instances of seizures, the impact of narcolepsy and sleep-related respiratory disorders. He does note:"*The pattern of violence against others is mostly an unconstructed violence against a bystander who may not be recognized by the wandering subject The most likely bystander, given the time these nocturnal episodes occur, is a caregiver or family member, often leading to a heart breaking situation for the perpetrator of the violent act.*" Siclari *et al* recently (2010) reviewed the violence in sleep literature [30]. They noted that apart from the NREM parasomnias (Confusional Arousals, Sleepwalking and Sleep Terror) and REM parasomnias (RBD) that epileptic conditions such as Nocturnal Paroxysmal Dystonia and Epileptic Nocturnal Wandering, Confusional States, Psychiatric dissociative states and malingering could also account for (apparently) sleep-related violence. They also listed numerous court cases which perhaps is less than desirable (see below) but amongst other topics usefully provided a summary distinguishing between arousal disorders and nocturnal seizures in nocturnal frontal lobe epilepsy. Ebrahim & Fenwick [31] provide the most comprehensive listing for differential diagnosis (see Table 2) and controversially use an alcohol provocation test in their sample case. Their work has led to some controversy [32-40].

Organic medical and neurologic disorders
Vascular
Mass lesions
Toxic/metabolic
Infectious (limbic encephalitis).
Central nervous system (CNS) trauma.
Seizure disorders e.g. partial complex seizures.
Nocturnal seizures
Narcolepsy and idiopathic hypersomnia.
Sleep apnoea.
Sleep deprivation.
Sleep schedule/circadian rhythm disorder (including jet-lag).
Psychogenic disorders (Dissociative states, Fugues. Multiple personality disorder)
Psychogenic amnesia.
Post-traumatic stress disorder.
Malingering.
Munchausen by proxy.

Table 2. Ebrahim & Fenwick provide a comprehensive list of possible aetiologies to aid differential diagnosis [31]

4. Forensic guidelines for sleep-related violence

In forensic psychiatry it not unusual to consider a behaviour in terms of predisposing (e.g. heredity), priming (e.g. sleep deprivation) and precipitating (e.g. touch) factors. Pressman in a series of papers has examined reviewed the literature to consider variables such as touch, sleep deprivation, febrile illness, etc. [37, 41] with a particular focus on sleep recording correlates [42] and alcohol [24, 38]. He has also questioned whether in cases that involve alcohol, whether the amnesia associated with the alleged event is caused by the putative parasomnia or is merely the result of an alcohol blackout [43] and whether the apparent association is a result of a methodological bias in the way the data has been collected (i.e. if a sleepwalker says they walk more often but are amnesic then how do they know, and how reliable is a third-party's information on the association) [24].

Feature	Violent behaviour	SRSBs	Comment
History	Corroborated	+	For violent behaviours there is usually a history of childhood sleepwalking or other deep sleep parasomnias. For adult onset there should also be some evidence in the clinical history or support from observers (ideally independent). For sexual behaviours previous bed partners may corroborate the behaviour.
Defendant asleep		+	There should be evidence that the defendant was asleep.
Asleep for how long	30 mins - two hours	?	For cases of violence it is rare for the behaviour to occur around the time of sleep onset. More usually around the time that deep sleep occurs (the first three hours of the night). For sexual behaviours - the behaviour may occur later in the night (as it may with sleepwalking - Mwenge et al, 2013 [44)]
Sleep exceptionally deep	Fatigue, drugs, alcohol, fever	?	Bonkalo[44] identifies this factor
Aroused/ (awoken)	Touch, etc	+	*cf [36, 44]*
Impulsive/short	Behaviours occurs on arousal	?	Most guidelines suggest durations of a few minutes to 30 minutes.
Victim accidental		?	The rarer form of sleep-related sexual assault is when the 'somnambulist' perambulates to the victim.
Amnesia	None, or marginal	?	Sexual 'RBD' (see Schenck et al 2007 review) [8]
Return to awareness	Incomprehension, possibly horror at act	?	In many cases both the victim and defendant remain asleep and the assault may not reported immediately.

Table 3. Forensic sleep guidelines [11, 12, 30, 31, 44, 46-49]

Guidelines as to how to assess these cases have been available at least since Bonkalo (1974) [44] reviewed the literature. His guidelines which had a strong focus on *Confusional Arousals* and cases of violence have been adopted and amended by various authors since. Table 4 summarises these guidelines. With minor variations these guidelines are the same.

For my own part before considering the guidelines that are available the questions that need to be answered are: 1) is the defendant capable of this behaviour whilst asleep (i.e. is there a compatible history) and not affected by confounding factors (e.g. medicines, drugs, alcohol, et) and 2) is the alleged behaviour compatible with a sleep-related disorder (i.e. a parasomnia)?

Sleepwalking – Simple behaviours turning into longer duration wandering?

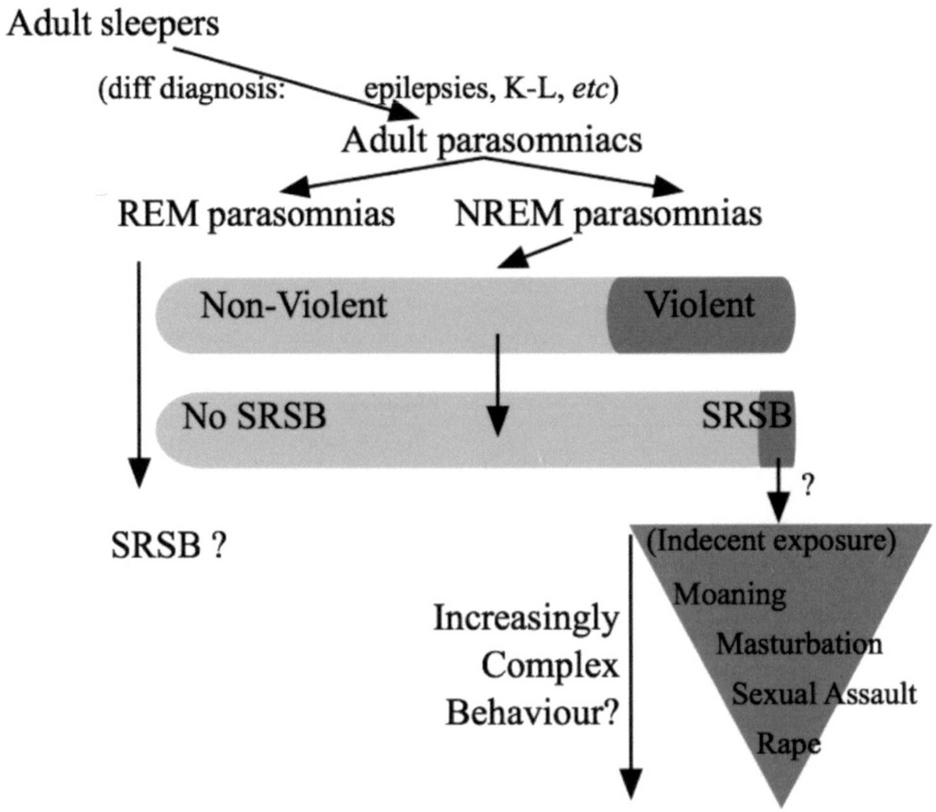

Figure 2. An illustration that attempts to show the decreasing incidence of a complex SRSB such as rape (though ejaculation is not noted).

4.1. Sleep-related sexual behaviour

ICDS3 lists SRSBs as a pathologic subtype under *Confusional Arousals* (A NREM parasomnia). However, not all SRSBs occur as NREM parasomnias (Table 5). SRSBs first emerged as a possible subtype of parasomnia with a description of masturbation by Wong [13]. This was

http://dx.doi.org/10.5772/59140

followed by case reports of sleep-related sexual abuse of children [50] and subsequently more reports from Shapiro [10] and Rosenfeld [49] with Guilleminault [12] providing the largest, substantive, well-investigated case series with Shapiro [11] running roughly parallel. Schenck et al [6] subsequently provide the first major review of the area.

•	Sleep sex, sexsomnia, sexual behaviour in sleep
•	Sleep sex moaning, sleep sex talking, sleep-sex shouting
•	Sleepsex snoring
•	Hypersexuality with Kleine-Levin syndrome;
•	Epileptic sleep sex/sexsomnia/SBS, sleep related sexual seizures
•	Epileptic sleep sex moaning, sleep sex talking, sleep sex shouting
•	Chronic, severe insomnia;
•	Restless legs syndrome (RLS)
•	Sexual hypnagogic or hypnopompic;
•	Sexual REM-onset dream attack
•	Cataplectic orgasm, peri-orgasmic cataplexy
•	Sleep exacerbation of persistent sexual arousal syndrome
•	Hypersexuality with sleep related painful erections (SRPE)
•	Hypersexuality with sleep related dissociative disorders
•	Hypersexuality during nocturnal awakenings
•	Nocturnal sexual delusions and hallucinations
(Terms used for searching for SRSBs in the published research literature by Schenk et al [6] for their 2007 review)	

Table 4. Sleep related abnormal sexual behaviours (alternate names)

It is notable that the largest number of cases was derived from patients suffering from Kleine-Levine Syndrome (78 cases), follow by parasomniacs [31] and sleep-related seizures (7 cases).

Schenck et al [6] note that neither the Kinsey [51, 52], apart from male nocturnal emissions, or Hite Reports [53, 54] note SRSBs. In the section on "Individual Variation, " Kinsey commented on the wide variety of human sexual behaviour which may have been a covert reference to nocturnal or sleep-related behaviour. They also note that their data, because of the sources contain cases that have led to criminal proceedings. Importantly they find that the greatest incidence of SRSBs is with patients suffering from Kleine-Levin syndrome, a rare disorder (probable incidence 1 in a million) characterised by periods of hypersomnia and mood changes, and with many patients suffering from hypersexuality and/or hyperphagia. Seventy-eight cases were reported. The next main group was the parasomnias-31 cases, followed by 7 cases of sleep-related seizures. Schenck et al [6] also question the existence of REM-related SRSBs or at least note there are no sleep laboratory confirmations of this behaviour and that the cases they reviewed did not involve dream-enactment. Parasomnia Overlap Disorder (a mixture of NREM and REM parasomnia was noted).

Kleine-Levin syndrome
Sleep related sexual seizures
Severe chronic insomnia
Restless legs syndrome
Narcolepsy
Sleep exacerbation of persistent sexual arousal syndrome
Sleep related painful erections and increased sexual activity
Sleep related dissociative disorders
Nocturnal psychotic disorders
Hypersexuality after nocturnal awakenings
Miscellaneous
(naps; [REM] sleep erections and sexual vulnerability; medication-induced states)

Table 5. Sleep Related Disorders and Abnormal Sexual behaviours and Experiences

It is perhaps surprising that the published clinical literature has relatively few SRSB case studies, given that an internet survey [55-57] ? The answer may lie in dream mentation work. Nielsen found that the prevalence of various behaviours particularly sexual behaviours apparently increased if respondents were asked specific questions about the behaviour; subjects did not readily reveal their sexual behaviour without being asked. Overall Nielsen noted that "females reported more speaking, crying, fear and smiling/laughing than did males; males reported more sexual arousal" [58].

4.2. Sleep-related sexual violence

Andersen *et al* (2007) [59] provide a slightly more focussed review than Shenck *et al*, 2007 [6] on SRSBs but include the main datasets provided by Guilleminault [12] and Shapiro [11]. The total number of cases cited was 40 (9 women). If the cases that were involved in criminal or other legal proceedings are excluded the number falls to 22 (7 women) ; if alcohol is then excluded there remain 17 cases (6 women). Further, if cases of multiple substance abuse and indecent exposure are removed that leaves a dataset of 15 (6 women). Of these there were 3 cases of sexual intercourse (men). Interaction between two individuals which is an assault without consent occurred with 7/9 men, and 1/6 women. Moaning was reported for 3/6 women and 1/10 men; masturbation 3/6 women and 2/10 men.

It is now becoming clear that slow wave sleep consists of not only different types of slow wave but these types have different functions [103-109]. It follows that when generalisations are

Variable	R&K 1968 [60]	AASM 2007 [61]	Comments	
Scoring page/ window length	15, 20 or 30 seconds	30 seconds (compulsory)	Originally sleep stages were scored on pages which consisted of 15-30 seconds data	
Stages	Wakefulness, stage 1 (drowsy), stage 2 (light), stage 3, stage 4, REM sleep, movement time.	Stages W, N1, N2, N3, and R	**Combinations and alternative names**: NREM = N1+N2+N3; REM sleep = Paradoxical sleep	
				Mental world
Wakefulness	EEG alpha activity for ≥50% of an epoch	Same (W)	Multiple variants	Awake (full range)
N3 **Deep sleep = Delta Sleep = SWS = Slow Wave Sleep, stages 3 and 4 combined.**	EEG slow-wave activity for ≥50% of the page for stage 4 sleep or ≥20% of the page for stage 3 sleep, 0.5-2.0 Hz and >75 µV	Same, except that stages 3 and 4 are combined to N3	Not all slow waves are the same. Some are very slow oscillations <1 Hz or classified according to different amplitudes	Nil or dark and threatening (usually associated with amnesia upon awakening)
N2 **Stage 2** **(light sleep)**	Sleep spindles or K-complexes; EEG slow-wave activity for <20% of the page	Same (N2)	Not all sleep spindles or K-complexes are the same	Identifies sleep onset in some systems.
N1 **Stage 1** **(drowsiness)**	Low-voltage, mixed-frequency activity; possibly slow eye movements; no sleep spindles or K-complexes; EEG alpha activity for <50% of the epoch	Same (N1)		Identifies sleep onset in some systems. Possible hallucinations
REM **REM sleep**	Low-voltage, mixed-frequency EEG activity; very low submental EMG activity; possible saw tooth EEG theta activity; >=1 rapid eye movement (unequivocal)	Same (R)	Phasic activity, sawtooth waves	Dreaming (full range of possible, nil, black & white, colour, etc). Dream incorporation, Dream enactment

AASM, American Academy of Sleep Medicine; EEG, electroencephalogram; EMG, electromyogram; R&K, Rechtschaffen and Kales [60].

Table 6. Showing classification rules and nomenclature of sleep staging systems.

made about deep sleep, those generalisations may not apply to all type of deep sleep. That degree of inaccuracy is below that usually required by courts that are seeking the truth. Spindles have the same problem [110-113].

The table is provided to enable comparison of older research with the new American Academy guidelines. That main point is that precisely what the sleep stages are is still a matter of research, debate and discussion. The original committee had difficulty in deciding on the stages (Oswald, personal communication, 1978 and others on the committee) and the 2007 still had similar problems. However it is notable that the professional sleep societies continue to monitor and refine the definitions (e.g. [62]). New 'stages' continue to be found, e.g. Koch et al [63]. For applied purposes like legal cases though the stages that cause most problems are REM and deep sleep. Further discussion in Idzikowski (2014) [64].

Sleep research and sleep medicine using electroencephalography ('brainwaves') as the primary measures grew with the discovery that 'dreaming' could be measured objectively [65]. Unfortunately, over time it turned out that the correlation between electrophysiological measures that lead to a particular classification of sleep stages was just a correlation (see Table 5 for definitions) ; dreaming generally occurs during REM but may occur in other stages, etc. Also, awkwardly both subjective appreciation, or behavioural responses do not directly map on to sleep stage. So in 'light sleep', (stage 2/N2) which is generally regarded as 'sleep' behavioural responses are still possible (depending on the time of night) [66].

The problem of identifying the stages accurately as indexed by the difficulties in producing automatic computer algorithms to do the staging and the disagreements between human scorers when sleep records are compared. Rosenberg et al, found sleep stage agreement averaged 82.6%. Agreement was highest for stage R sleep with stages N2 and W approaching the same level. Scoring agreement for stage N3 sleep was 67.4% and was lowest for stage N1 at 63.0% (the stages that are important with regard to NREM parasomnias. Scorers had particular difficulty with the last epoch of stage W before sleep onset, the first epoch of stage N2 after stage N1 and the first epoch of stage R after stage N2. Discrimination between stages N2 and N3 was particularly difficult for scorers [62].

In addition to compartmentalising sleep into page lengths of 20-30 seconds there have been other attempts to quantify sleep that are less reliant on page size and that may be important in the definition of sleep, deep sleep and sleepwalking. For example, spectral analysis (looking at the frequency domains) [67, 68, 69, 70] and Cyclic Alternating Pattern CAP [69].

In humans sleep has a 90 minute cyclicity [71, 72], and in normal individuals there is a preponderance of deep (N3) sleep early in the night, with progressively more REM sleep occurring late in the sleep period. The 90 minute cycle is punctuated with REM sleep and possibly wakefulness. Deep sleep is homeostatically controlled as is REM sleep, but REM sleep also has a circadian component with more REM sleep occurring in the morning.

It is important to note that when the hypothalamic and lower brain sleep centres are most active, the wake centres are generally quiescent. The interplay between the two orchestrates some of the changes seen in the brain. Loss of conscious awareness occurs some time during stage 2 when functional MRI signals decrease in the tale thalamic and hypothalamic regions, the cingulate cortex, right insula, nearby temporal regions, the inferior parietal lobules and the inferior/middle frontal gyri [78]. Bassetti *et al* [79] have observed in one subject during sleepwalking that a disassociation between an activation in thalamocingulate pathways

http://dx.doi.org/10.5772/59140

AREA	DEEP SLEEP	REM SLEEP
Lateral frontal cortex	↓	↓
Medial prefrontal + orbitofrontal cortex		↑ ↓
Lateral parietal cortex	↓	↓
Medial parietal cortex +precuneus	↓	↓
Temporal-occipital cortices	↑	↑
Anterior cingulate cortex		↑
Medial temporal lobe, hippocampal regions, amygdala		↑
Thalamus	↓	↑
Basal ganglia	↓	
Pons, midbrain	↓	
Cerebellum	↓	

Table 7. Provides an overview of brain imaging studies that show both the decreases and increases in brain activity during the major sleep stages [73-77].

coupled with deactivation of thalamocortical arousal systems is associated with sleepwalking. It is almost important to note though that within cortical regions there can be both increases and decreases of activity within "sleep" which are presumed to reflect local energy requirements [80, 81]

Sleep is an orchestrated state with hypothalamic centres strongly controlling which areas of brain remain active and which become quiescent-see Table 7. Diminution of activity in areas such as the prefrontal cortex underpin the scientific arguments that the brain centres that might be involved in the determining whether a behaviour is 'right or wrong', appropriate or not are not active. That coupled with evidence from sleep deprivation work that points to degraded moral judgement with sleep loss [82].

Whilst this section and sleep classifications describe sleep states as mutually exclusive, in reality they are not. The stages are an amalgam of different physiological signs that have been lumped together as stages (by committee and consensus). That does not mean that all aspects associated with a particular stage will necessarily remain within that stage. For example a penile erection which is usually associated with REM sleep may continue, for a period of time, into light sleep or wakefulness? Moreover, there is still debate as to what the functional significance of sleep stages. Pharmacological disassociations have occasionally been noted, e.g. changes in deep sleep duration without apparent impact on waking function [83]. Mahowald and Schenck [84] describe the extreme states of wakefulness whilst apparently asleep (according to electrophysiological characteristics). Mahowald and Schenck identify the three basic states of being as wakefulness, NREM sleep and REM sleep.

5. Alcohol and sleep

Bonkalo notes alcohol amongst factors that may increase deep sleep and thus facilitate violent confusional arousals [44]. ICSD3 explicitly states [17] "... Disorders of arousal should not be diagnosed in the presence of alcohol intoxication. The behavior of the alcohol-intoxicated individual may superficially resemble that of the sleepwalker. ..." This is within a section on differential diagnosis but it also may have an undue impact in the forensic area. Why this sort of policy statement should be placed in a scientific document is not entirely clear. It is correct to note that there are difficulties, but an instance of a behaviour that may occur without alcohol could be repeated within sleep, irrespective of whether alcohol is present or not? However, there is confusion in the literature as alcohol has been suggested as a priming factor, partly on the basis of self-reports, rejected by Pressman *et al* [24] because of recall bias, and partly as early hypotheses noted that: 1) deep sleep is associated with sleepwalking, 2) alcohol facilitates deep sleep (not currently, wholly accepted) and 3) they hypothesis, so alcohol must promote sleepwalking? No formal experiments have been published either refuting or accepting this hypothesis and in fact given the reported complex effects of alcohol on sleep [36] and the variables involved, e.g. Carskadon and colleagues [85-88], it may be quite some time before an adequate experiment on sleepwalkers is conducted. Answering the question as to how alcohol might affect sexual response [89, 90] during sleep exacerbates the complexities.

6. Wakefulness and violence

Sleep and wakefulness are two sides of the same coin. Sleep-related legal cases need to be balanced by considering what can happen when a person is awake. Humans are inherently a violent species, both in terms of physical aggression and aggression directed sexually [91]. Sleep-related violence has only a loose overlap with WHO's typology of violence. The overlap is interpersonal violence which may be physical or sexual. It is unknown whether self-directed violence in the form of suicidal behaviour occurs during sleep as it is assumed that sleepwalkers who have perished did not intend to commit suicide. The links between violent assaults and wakefulness are broad and will not be considered here.

6.1. Wakefulness and sexual violence

There are multiple risk factors that increase the risk of a man committing rape. These include individual factors such as alcohol and drug use; coercive sexual fantasies, attitudes and beliefs supportive of sexual violence; impulsive and antisocial tendencies; preference for impersonal sex; hostility towards women; history of sexual abuse as a child; witnessing family violence as a child. Additionally, relationship factors (e.g. associating with sexually aggressive and delinquent peers), community factors (e.g. lack of employment opportunities, general tolerance of sexual assault within the community) and societal factors (e.g. societal norms supportive of sexual violence, male superiority and sexual entitlement). Conservative estimates suggest that at least 25 percent of American women have been assaulted in adolescence or adulthood and that 18 percent have been raped. Furthermore, at least 20 percent of American men report having perpetrated sexual assault and 5 percent report having committed rape [92].

In the United Kingdom (North London, 1993) 6% assaulted in the past 12 months, and 23% attempted or completed forced sex by an intimate partner [93, 94]. The comparable figures for the U.S. are 0.7% and 7.7% but these may be skewed as the sample group did not include women who had been in a relationship [91].

6.2. Alcohol and sexual violence

The biological links between alcohol and violence are complex. Even the impact of alcohol on sexual potency needs further research as results currently still need clarification-e.g. high doses of alcohol which might render some men impotent do not appear to have the same effects on rapists [95]. Alcohol does though have a disinhibiting role in sexual assaults, it reduces inhibitions, clouds judgements and impairs ability to interpret cues [91]. As lack of reporting causes a problem in identifying the precise incidence of alcohol being associated with rape, the estimates are similar to violent crime in general and range between 34-74% [92]. The role of alcohol is complex [96].

7. Discussion

It is perhaps not surprising that there are calls for more considered opinions and further research into the whole area of sleep-related violence, let alone sleep-related sexual violence [97]. Extrapolating what is known about parasomnias, given the limited evidence base, which at best is still only at the data-collection phase, to applied situations such as legal cases have to be fraught. There are varying degrees of certainty with respect to what we know: 1) in NREM deep sleep, associated with short-duration somnambulism (within the confines of one sleep cycle), there is a) limited or fragmentary connection with the external world, b) some mental activity that may be concordant with behaviour, and c) behaviours including ambulation that are relatively simple. 2) It is not clear, particularly with longer duration, more complex behaviours, whether deep sleep continues, or whether sleep either moves into a more wakeful but disassociated state, or to drowsiness and/or light sleep but still possibly in a disassociated state. 3) The normal cyclicity of sleep is disturbed. The main hypotheses dealing with sleep control posit an interaction between a sleep homeostat and the circadian system. There is curiously little evidence that the circadian system is involved, other than most (if not all) NREM parasomnias occur at night? However, circadian displacement is being increasingly implicated [115]. The homeostat increases the pressure for sleep, particularly deep sleep, in parallel with the duration of prior wakefulness. However, in sleepwalkers this system appears to be faulty [25], with their deep sleep being more broken with arousals and wakefulness (which could be a circadian system effect, with circadian time being affected by the sleep deprivation?).With SRSBs there is a range of possibilities ranging from simple caresses to sexual intercourse, all of which may lead to legal action if occurring inappropriately and without consent. The current database of recorded sexual activity is sparse and what there is has been with consenting adults dressed for sleep. Apart from sexual intercourse rape may involve unclothing a possibly unfamiliar victim, and also possibly in unfamiliar circumstances. Whilst erection and ejaculation are underpinned by primarily reflexive mechanisms, more complex control is required to achieve full intercourse with ejaculation.

It is perhaps not surprising that the emerging (sub-?) speciality of 'forensic sleep' or 'forensic sleep medicine', given the limited database, ambiguities over the function of sleep or its staging, that the area has little theoretical underpinning. Perhaps though the time has come to start theorising or creating testable models against which to run hypotheses? This has already started thought at a basic level. Cramer Bornemann and Mahowald [114] leaning on the concept of central pattern generators provide some ideas as to how simple, reflexive and instinctive behaviours may arise in humans during sleep. Zadra et al [25] consider the existing evidence to assemble a model describing somnambulistic behaviour. This suggests that there are two main dimensions to sleepwalking: a dysfunctional "deep sleep" system, and b) a dysfunctional arousal (wake-promoting) system.

7.1. What can sleep science & sleep medicine tell the law?

Sleep research has identified various stages of sleep though there are still debates as to scoring of the stages and their functional significance. As noted earlier, there are also ambiguities as to when sleep onset actually occurs and very little work on what cognitive capacity remains-(insight, problem-solving, etc.) (dreams are a special case, where a mixture of brain imaging and self-report identities what brain regions appear inactive, and provides more information e.g. reduced firing in the locus coeuruleus would lead external stimuli having less impact on attention-which may account for a dream narrative incorporating external stimuli as opposed to breaking the narrative (and awakening the subject?) [98].

For forensic work the main issues are how (particular stages of) sleep can affect cognitive capacity, and control of behaviour. The impact of sleep deprivation and sleep restriction on waking sleepiness and cognitive capacity is not dealt with in this chapter. This needs further consideration as the complexity of behaviour in an alleged crime is important, e.g. what capacity is required for a defendant to appreciate consent, what capacity is required for a 'sleeping?' rapist to seek out and locate a victim? At which point does apparent capacity preclude the possibility that the defendant is in fact not asleep (they may be awake but may be in a different state, a disassociated state of some sort (not necessarily sleep-related)).

In normal REM sleep the muscles are paralysed so movement is more or less impossible. However penile tumescence is normal and in some circumstances the meaning of an erection can be misconstrued (leading to legal action). Given that sleep is a usually coordinated state the tumescence would normally subside prior to or when entering other stages, like wakefulness (with the possibility of sleep inertia) or drowsiness or light or even deep sleep. At sleep onset, the precise determination of the onset of mental sleep is unclear, occurring sometime during N2 (light sleep). 'Wet dreams' are not regarded as pathological, when ejaculation occurs during [REM?] sleep. Clearly, some movements occur during sleep to maintain comfort (either avoiding pain or maintaining an appropriate temperature, etc), but even these if someone is sleeping nearby, these movements may accidentally impact on the other sleeper which in some circumstances can lead to complaints of assault.

Sleep medicine can describe somnambulistic episodes only roughly (virtually no helpful home recordings), quite roughly-both duration and timing of episodes are subject to dispute. Consider Mwenge et al's sleepwalker whose latest episode was 06.45-using home recordings [45].

7.2. What can the law tell sleep science and medicine?

Judicial systems have had to manage sleep-related states considerably a lot longer than the time that sleep science and medicine have existed (considerably longer than the Royal College of Psychiatrists!). Understanding the nuances where they are not policy driven can be a useful area to explore. Unfortunately though, reliable data as to individual cases is rarely available. Media misreporting is common. Attention demanding headlines or misreporting by legal correspondents creates difficulties that may ultimately influence professional opinions and misguide the opinions experts may give in court. Furthermore, publishing of case studies is fraught with difficulty if reference is made to court proceedings. Case material acquired during a court case is not in the public domain. A defendant whether convicted or not retains their human rights and although the confidentiality between practitioner and client is broken in relation to the court, that does not necessarily (arguable) make the material available to the public domain.

8. Future agendas

Basic science research: arousal thresholds, sensory/cognitive processing capability, classical/ operant conditioning potential. Better models of human sexual behaviour. Development of home recording equipment (video, ambulatory systems (e.g. like the Zeo [99-102]. There is also a need for better models of describing the relationship of sleep and wakefulness with cognition and behaviour (the subject of another paper).

Clinical science research: improved classifications systems; the need to distinguish between somnambulism, sleep inertia and disassociated states.

Forensic: Some definition of standards and methodologies driven not only by a reaction to legal needs but also by consideration of basic pathophysiology. The effect of alcohol needs to be explored both in a laboratory and non-laboratory setting (initially outside of a legal context).

Legal: Reform and uniformity across jurisdictions with respect to insanity and automatism laws. Ideally a mechanism to record accurately court proceedings and the data associated with these cases, so that it is possible to court cases as data.

9. Conclusion

This essay focused on NREM parasomnias that might lead to SRSB that in turn might lead to legal proceedings. A considerable amount of work needs to be done so that expert opinion in court is based on science that has substantive forensic value.

Acknowledgements

Former colleagues of Sleep Medicine Centre Ltd (Edinburgh Sleep Centre-Heriot Row and the London Sleep Centre – Harley Street) especially Ewan Crawford, Lizzie Hill, Stevie Williams, Heather Engleman, Laura Bolton, Christine Auld, Susan Fifer, Mario Alfredo Parra-Rodriguez, Marios Kittenis, and Elvina Gountouna.

Prisons: HMPs Belmarsh, Swansea, Peterborough, Holloway, Durham, Exeter and Edinburgh (at the Edinburgh Sleep Centre – Heriot Row)

Author details

Chris Idzikowski*

Address all correspondence to: chris.idzikowski@neuronic.com

Innis Court, Holywood House, Holywood, Co Down, BT18 9HF, Northern Ireland

References

[1] Umanath S, Sarezky D, Finger S. Sleepwalking through history: Medicine, arts, and courts of law. J Hist Neurosci 2011, Oct; 20 (4); 253-76.

[2] Petrain DE. An english translation of john william polidoris (1815) medical dissertation on oneirodynia (somnambulism). European Romantic Review 2010; 21 (6); 775-88.

[3] Ekirch AR, Shneerson JM. Nineteenth-Century sleep violence cases: A historical view. Sleep Med Clin 2011, Dec; 6 (4); 483-91.

[4] Rubin G. The" political economy" of sex. Feminist Anthropology: A Reader 2009:87.

[5] Kompanje EJO. 'The devil lay upon her and held her down' hypnagogic hallucinations and sleep paralysis described by the dutch physician isbrand van diemerbroeck (1609–1674) in 1664. J Sleep Res 2008; 17 (4); 464-7.

[6] Schenck CH, Arnulf I, Mahowald MW. Sleep and sex: What can go wrong? A review of the literature on sleep related disorders and abnormal sexual behaviors and experiences. Sleep 2007, Jun; 30 (6); 683-702.

[7] Hardy T. Tess of the d'urbervilles. New York: Nelson Doubleday; 1891 f.

[8] Bowden P. Sleepwalking and indecent exposure. Med Sci Law 1991, Oct; 31 (4); 359.

[9] Buchanan A. Sleepwalking and indecent exposure. Med Sci Law 1991, Jan; 31 (1); 38-40.

[10] Shapiro CM, Fedoroff JP, Trajanovic NN. Sexual behavior in sleep: A newly described parasomnia. Sleep Res 1996; 25:367.

[11] Shapiro CM, Trajanovic NN, Fedoroff JP. Sexsomnia--a new parasomnia? Can J Psychiatry 2003, Jun; 48 (5); 311-7.

[12] Guilleminault C, Moscovitch A, Yuen K, Poyares D. Atypical sexual behavior during sleep. Psychosom Med 2002; 64 (2); 328-36.

[13] Wong KE. Masturbation during sleep--a somnambulistic variant? Singapore Med J 1986, Dec; 27 (6); 542-3.

[14] Fenwick P. Sleep and sexual offending. Med Sci Law 1996, Apr; 36 (2); 122-34.

[15] Medicine AAOS. International classification of sleep disorders, 3rd edition. Darien, IL: American Academy Of Sleep Medicine; 2014f.

[16] Eastman N. Psychiatric, psychological, and legal models of man. Int J Law Psychiatry 1992; 15 (2); 157-69.

[17] ICSD nrem-related parasomnias. In: International Classification of Sleep Disorders. American Academy of Sleep Medicine, ; 2014g. p. 228-39.

[18] Pressman MR, Meyer TJ, Kendrick-Mohamed J, Figueroa WG, Greenspon LW, Peterson DD. Night terrors in an adult precipitated by sleep apnea. Sleep 1995, Nov; 18 (9); 773-5.

[19] Iranzo A, Santamaría J. Severe obstructive sleep apnea/hypopnea mimicking REM sleep behavior disorder. Sleep 2005, Feb; 28 (2); 203-6.

[20] Ohayon MM, Priest RG, Caulet M, Guilleminault C. Hypnagogic and hypnopompic hallucinations: Pathological phenomena? Br J Psychiatry 1996, Oct; 169 (4); 459-67.

[21] Ohayon MM. Prevalence of hallucinations and their pathological associations in the general population. Psychiatry Res 2000, Dec 27; 97 (2-3); 153-64.

[22] Hublin C, Kaprio J, Partinen M, Koskenvuo M. Sleeptalking in twins: Epidemiology and psychiatric comorbidity. Behav Genet 1998, Jul; 28 (4); 289-98.

[23] Lopez R, Jaussent I, Scholz S, Bayard S, Montplaisir J, Dauvilliers Y. Functional impairment in adult sleepwalkers: A case-control study. Sleep 2013, Mar; 36 (3); 345-51.

[24] Pressman MR. Sleepwalking, amnesia, comorbid conditions and triggers: Effects of recall and other methodological biases. Sleep 2013, Nov; 36 (11); 1757-8.

[25] Zadra A, Desautels A, Petit D, Montplaisir J. Somnambulism: Clinical aspects and pathophysiological hypotheses. Lancet Neurol 2013, Mar; 12 (3); 285-94.

[26] Moldofsky H, Gilbert R, Lue FA, MacLean AW. Sleep-related violence. Sleep 1995, Nov; 18 (9); 731-9.

[27] Ohayon MM, Caulet M, Priest RG. Violent behavior during sleep. J Clin Psychiatry 1997, Aug; 58 (8); 369-76; quiz 377.

[28] Ohayon MM, Schenck CH. Violent behavior during sleep: Prevalence, comorbidity and consequences. Sleep Med 2010, Oct; 11 (9); 941-6.

[29] Guilleminault C, Leger D, Philip P, Ohayon MM. Nocturnal wandering and violence: Review of a sleep clinic population. J Forensic Sci 1998, Jan; 43 (1); 158-63.

[30] Siclari F, Khatami R, Urbaniok F, Nobili L, Mahowald MW, Schenck CH, et al. Violence in sleep. Brain 2010, Dec; 133 (Pt 12); 3494-509.

[31] Ebrahim O, Fenwick P. Sleep-related automatism and the law. Med Sci Law 2008, Apr 1; 48 (2); 124-36.

[32] Pressman MR. Alcohol does not increase slow wave sleep. Alcohol Clin Exp Res 2012, Aug; 36 (8); 1474; author reply 1475.

[33] Pressman MR, Mahowald MW, Cramer–Bornemann M. Reply to Ebrahim and Fenwick. Sleep Med Rev 2007, Jun; 11 (3); 244-7.

[34] Mahowald MW, Schenck CH, Cramer Bornemann MA. Response to Ebrahim and Fenwick. Sleep Med Rev 2007, Jun; 11 (3); 247.

[35] Ebrahim I, Fenwick PB. Response to pressman: "Factors that predispose, prime and precipitate NREM parasomnias in adults: Clinical and forensic implications" sleep med. Rev. 2007; 11:5-9. Sleep Med Rev 2007, Jun; 11 (3); 241-3; author reply 244-7.

[36] Ebrahim IO, Shapiro CM, Williams AJ, Fenwick PB. Alcohol and sleep I: Effects on normal sleep. Alcohol Clin Exp Res 2013, Apr; 37 (4); 539-49.

[37] Pressman MR. Factors that predispose, prime and precipitate NREM parasomnias in adults: Clinical and forensic implications. Sleep Med Rev 2007, Feb; 11 (1); 5-30; discussion 31-3.

[38] Pressman MR, Mahowald MW, Schenck CH, Bornemann MC. Alcohol-induced sleepwalking or confusional arousal as a defense to criminal behavior: A review of scientific evidence, methods and forensic considerations. J Sleep Res 2007, Jun; 16 (2); 198-212.

[39] Pressman MR, Schenck CH, Mahowald MW, Bornemann MC. Sleep science in the courtroom. J Forensic Leg Med 2007, Feb; 14 (2); 108-11; author reply 111-3, discussion 114-8.

[40] Ebrahim I, Fenwick P. Letter to the editor re: Pressman et al. Alcohol-induced sleepwalking or confusional arousal as a defense to criminal behavior: A review of scientific evidence, methods and forensic considerations. J. Sleep res. (2007) 16, 198-212. J Sleep Res 2008, Dec; 17 (4); 470-2; author reply 473-4.

[41] Pressman MR. Disorders of arousal from sleep and violent behavior: The role of physical contact and proximity. Sleep 2007, Aug; 30 (8); 1039-47.

[42] Pressman MR. Hypersynchronous delta sleep EEG activity and sudden arousals from slow-wave sleep in adults without a history of parasomnias: Clinical and forensic implications. Sleep 2004, Jun 15; 27 (4); 706-10.

[43] Pressman MR, Caudill DS. Alcohol-induced blackout as a criminal defense or mitigating factor: An evidence-based review and admissibility as scientific evidence. J Forensic Sci 2013, Jul; 58 (4); 932-40.

[44] Bonkalo A. Impulsive acts and confusional states during incomplete arousal from sleep: Criminological and forensic implications. Psychiatr Q 1974; 48 (3); 400-9.

[45] Mwenge B, Brion A, Uguccioni G, Arnulf I. Sleepwalking: Long-term home video monitoring. Sleep Med 2013, Nov; 14 (11); 1226-8.

[46] Buchanan PR. Sleep sex. Sleep Med Clin 2011, Dec; 6 (4); 417-28.

[47] Ebrahim I, Wilson W, Marks R, Peacock KW, Fenwick P. Violence, sleepwalking and the criminal law: (1) the medical aspects. Criminal Law Review 2005:601-13.

[48] Mahowald MW, Bundlie SR, Hurwitz TD, Schenck CH. Sleep violence--forensic science implications: Polygraphic and video documentation. J Forensic Sci 1990, Mar; 35 (2); 413-32.

[49] Rosenfeld DS, Elhajjar AJ. Sleepsex: A variant of sleepwalking. Arch Sex Behav 1998, Jun; 27 (3); 269-78.

[50] Hurwitz TD, Mahowald MW, Schluter JL. Sleep-related sexual abuse of children. Sleep Res 1989; 18:246.

[51] Kinsey AC. Sexual behavior in the human female. Indiana University Press; 1953f.

[52] Kinsey AC, Pomeroy WB, Martin CE. Sexual behavior in the human male. 1948.

[53] Hite S. The hite report: A nationwide study of female sexuality. Seven Stories Press; 2004h.

[54] Hite S. The hite report on male sexuality. Knopf New York; 1981i.

[55] Mangan MA. A phenomenology of problematic sexual behavior occurring in sleep. Arch Sex Behav 2004, Jun; 33 (3); 287-93.

[56] Mangan MA, Reips UD. Sleep, sex, and the web: Surveying the difficult-to-reach clinical population suffering from sexsomnia. Behav Res Methods 2007, May; 39 (2); 233-6.

[57] Trajanovic NN, Mangan M, Shapiro CM. Sexual behaviour in sleep: An internet survey. Soc Psychiatry Psychiatr Epidemiol 2007, Dec; 42 (12); 1024-31.

[58] Nielsen T, Svob C, Kuiken D. Dream-enacting behaviors in a normal population. Sleep 2009, Dec; 32 (12); 1629-36.

[59] Andersen ML, Poyares D, Alves RS, Skomro R, Tufik S. Sexsomnia: Abnormal sexual behavior during sleep. Brain Res Rev 2007, Dec; 56 (2); 271-82.

[60] Rechtschaffen A, Kales A. A manual of standardized terminology, technique and scoring system for sleep stages of human sleep. NIH publication no. 204. Washington DC: US Government Printing Office; 1968k.

[61] Medicine AAOS, Iber C. The AASM manual for the scoring of sleep and associated events: Rules, terminology and technical specifications. American Academy of Sleep Medicine; 2007l.

[62] Rosenberg RS, Van Hout S. The american academy of sleep medicine inter-scorer reliability program: Sleep stage scoring. J Clin Sleep Med 2013, Jan 15; 9 (1); 81-7.

[63] Koch H, Christensen JA, Frandsen R, Zoetmulder M, Arvastson L, Christensen SR, et al. Automatic sleep classification using a data-driven topic model reveals latent sleep states. J Neurosci Methods 2014, Jul 9; 235C:130-7.

[64] Idzikowski C. The pharmacology of human sleep, a work in progress? Curr Opin Pharmacol 2014, Feb; 14:90-6.

[65] Aserinksy E, Kleitman N. Regularly occurring periods of eye motility, and concomitant phenomena, during sleep. Science 1953, Sep 4; 118 (3062); 273-4.

[66] Ogilvie RD, Wilkinson RT, Allison S. The detection of sleep onset: Behavioral, physiological, and subjective convergence. Sleep 1989, Oct; 12 (5); 458-74.

[67] Guilleminault C, Poyares D, Aftab FA, Palombini L, Abat F. Sleep and wakefulness in somnambulism: A spectral analysis study. J Psychosom Res 2001, Aug; 51 (2); 411-6.

[68] Pilon M, Zadra A, Joncas S, Montplaisir J. Hypersynchronous delta waves and somnambulism: Brain topography and effect of sleep deprivation. Sleep 2006, Jan; 29 (1); 77-84.

[69] Guilleminault C. Hypersynchronous slow delta, cyclic alternating pattern and sleepwalking. Sleep 2006, Jan; 29 (1); 14-5.

[70] Guilleminault C, Kirisoglu C, da Rosa AC, Lopes C, Chan A. Sleepwalking, a disorder of NREM sleep instability. Sleep Med 2006, Mar; 7 (2); 163-70.

[71] Dijk DJ. Regulation and functional correlates of slow wave sleep. J Clin Sleep Med 2009, Apr 15; 5 (2 Suppl); S6-15.

[72] Kishi A, Yasuda H, Matsumoto T, Inami Y, Horiguchi J, Tamaki M, et al. NREM sleep stage transitions control ultradian REM sleep rhythm. Sleep 2011, Oct; 34 (10); 1423-32.

[73] Braun AR, Balkin TJ, Wesenten NJ, Carson RE, Varga M, Baldwin P, et al. Regional cerebral blood flow throughout the sleep-wake cycle. An H2 (15) O PET study. Brain 1997, Jul; 120 (Pt 7); 1173-97.

[74] Maquet P, Péters J, Aerts J, Delfiore G, Degueldre C, Luxen A, Franck G. Functional neuroanatomy of human rapid-eye-movement sleep and dreaming. Nature 1996, Sep 12; 383 (6596); 163-6.

[75] Maquet P, Degueldre C, Delfiore G, Aerts J, Péters JM, Luxen A, Franck G. Functional neuroanatomy of human slow wave sleep. J Neurosci 1997, Apr 15; 17 (8); 2807-12.

[76] Maquet P. Positron emission tomography studies of sleep and sleep disorders. J Neurol 1997, Apr; 244 (4 Suppl 1); S23-8.

[77] Maquet P, Phillips C. Functional brain imaging of human sleep. J Sleep Res 1998; 7 Suppl 1:42-7.

[78] Kaufmann C, Wehrle R, Wetter TC, Holsboer F, Auer DP, Pollmächer T, Czisch M. Brain activation and hypothalamic functional connectivity during human non-rapid eye movement sleep: An EEG/fmri study. Brain 2006, Mar; 129 (Pt 3); 655-67.

[79] Bassetti C, Vella S, Donati F, Wielepp P, Weder B. SPECT during sleepwalking. Lancet 2000, Aug 5; 356 (9228); 484-5.

[80] Terzaghi M, Sartori I, Tassi L, Didato G, Rustioni V, LoRusso G, et al. Evidence of dissociated arousal states during NREM parasomnia from an intracerebral neurophysiological study. Sleep 2009, Mar; 32 (3); 409-12.

[81] Dang-Vu TT, Schabus M, Desseilles M, Sterpenich V, Bonjean M, Maquet P. Functional neuroimaging insights into the physiology of human sleep. Sleep 2010, Dec; 33 (12); 1589-603.

[82] Killgore WD, Killgore DB, Day LM, Li C, Kamimori GH, Balkin TJ. The effects of 53 hours of sleep deprivation on moral judgment. Sleep 2007, Mar; 30 (3); 345-52.

[83] Idzikowski C, Mills FJ, Glennard R. 5-Hydroxytryptamine-2 antagonist increases human slow wave sleep. Brain Res 1986, Jul 16; 378 (1); 164-8.

[84] Mahowald MW, Schenck CH. Status dissociatus--a perspective on states of being. Sleep 1991, Feb; 14 (1); 69-79.

[85] Rupp TL, Acebo C, Seifer R, Carskadon MA. Effects of a moderate evening alcohol dose. II: Performance. Alcohol Clin Exp Res 2007, Aug; 31 (8); 1365-71.

[86] Rupp TL, Acebo C, Van Reen E, Carskadon MA. Effects of a moderate evening alcohol dose. I: Sleepiness. Alcohol Clin Exp Res 2007, Aug; 31 (8); 1358-64.

[87] Van Reen E, Rupp TL, Acebo C, Seifer R, Carskadon MA. Biphasic effects of alcohol as a function of circadian phase. Sleep 2013, Jan; 36 (1); 137-45.

[88] Van Reen E, Tarokh L, Rupp TL, Seifer R, Carskadon MA. Does timing of alcohol administration affect sleep? Sleep 2011, Feb; 34 (2); 195-205.

[89] George WH, Stoner SA. Understanding acute alcohol effects on sexual behavior. Annu Rev Sex Res 2000; 11:92-124.

[90] George WH, Cue Davis K, Schraufnagel TJ, Norris J, Heiman JR, Schacht RL, et al. Later that night: Descending alcohol intoxication and men's sexual arousal. Am J Mens Health 2008, Mar; 2 (1); 76-86.

[91] Krug EG, Mercy JA, Dahlberg LL, Zwi AB. The world report on violence and health. The Lancet 2002; 360 (9339); 1083-8.

[92] Abbey A, Zawacki T, Buck PO, Clinton AM, McAuslan P. Alcohol and sexual assault. Alcohol Research and Health 2001; 25 (1); 43-51.

[93] Mooney J. The hidden figure: Domestic violence in north london. Middlesex University, School of Sociology and Social Policy; 1993ae.

[94] Lancet Editorial. Opening the door on gender-based violence. Lancet 2012, Aug 25; 380 (9843); 703.

[95] The effects of alcohol on penile erection. Electronic ed. New York: Routledge; 2014ad.

[96] Johnson SA. Understanding the role of alcohol during rape: The perfect storm of attention, emotion, & expectancies. International Journal of Emergency Mental Health and Human Resilience 2014; 16 (1); 30-8.

[97] Morrison I, Rumbold JM, Riha RL. Medicolegal aspects of complex behaviours arising from the sleep period: A review and guide for the practising sleep physician. Sleep Med Rev 2014, Jun; 18 (3); 249-60.

[98] Maquet P, Ruby P, Maudoux A, Albouy G, Sterpenich V, Dang-Vu T, et al. Human cognition during REM sleep and the activity profile within frontal and parietal cortices: A reappraisal of functional neuroimaging data. In: ; 2005ag. p. 219-595.

[99] Gumenyuk V, Roth T, Korzyukov O, Jefferson C, Bowyer S, Drake CL. Habitual short sleep impacts frontal switch mechanism in attention to novelty. Sleep 2011, Dec; 34 (12); 1659-70.

[100] Marshall JC, Malerba JR, Schroeder JA. Use of personal EEG monitors in a behavioral neuroscience course to investigate natural setting sleep patterns and the factors affecting them in college students. J Undergrad Neurosci Educ 2011; 10 (1); A65-70.

[101] Shambroom JR, Fábregas SE, Johnstone J. Validation of an automated wireless system to monitor sleep in healthy adults. J Sleep Res 2012, Apr; 21 (2); 221-30.

[102] Griessenberger H, Heib DP, Kunz AB, Hoedlmoser K, Schabus M. Assessment of a wireless headband for automatic sleep scoring. Sleep Breath 2013, May; 17 (2); 747-52.

[103] Dang-Vu TT, Schabus M, Desseilles M, Albouy G, Boly M, Darsaud A, et al. Spontaneous neural activity during human slow wave sleep. Proc Natl Acad Sci U S A 2008, Sep 30; 105 (39); 15160-5.

[104] Mongrain V, Carrier J, Paquet J, Bélanger-Nelson E, Dumont M. Morning and evening-type differences in slow waves during NREM sleep reveal both trait and state-dependent phenotypes. PLoS One 2011; 6 (8); e22679.

[105] Feinberg I, de Bie E, Davis NM, Campbell IG. Topographic differences in the adolescent maturation of the slow wave EEG during NREM sleep. Sleep 2011, Mar; 34 (3); 325-33.

[106] Viola AU, Chellappa SL, Archer SN, Pugin F, Götz T, Dijk DJ, Cajochen C. Interindividual differences in circadian rhythmicity and sleep homeostasis in older people: Effect of a PER3 polymorphism. Neurobiol Aging 2012, May; 33 (5); 1010.e17-27.

[107] Mistlberger R, Bergmann B, Rechtschaffen A. Period-amplitude analysis of rat electroencephalogram: Effects of sleep deprivation and exercise. Sleep 1987, Dec; 10 (6); 508-22.

[108] Carrier J, Viens I, Poirier G, Robillard R, Lafortune M, Vandewalle G, et al. Sleep slow wave changes during the middle years of life. Eur J Neurosci 2011, Feb; 33 (4); 758-66.

[109] Saletin JM, van der Helm E, Walker MP. Structural brain correlates of human sleep oscillations. Neuroimage 2013, Dec; 83:658-68.

[110] Schabus M, Dang-Vu TT, Heib DP, Boly M, Desseilles M, Vandewalle G, et al. The fate of incoming stimuli during NREM sleep is determined by spindles and the phase of the slow oscillation. Front Neurol 2012; 3:40.

[111] Ruch S, Markes O, Duss SB, Oppliger D, Reber TP, Koenig T, et al. Sleep stage II contributes to the consolidation of declarative memories. Neuropsychologia 2012, Aug; 50 (10); 2389-96.

[112] Astori S, Wimmer RD, Lüthi A. Manipulating sleep spindles--expanding views on sleep, memory, and disease. Trends Neurosci 2013, Dec; 36 (12); 738-48.

[113] Thomas Andrillon YNRJSFFCCGTIF. Sleep spindles in humans: Insights from intracranial EEG and unit recordings. The Journal of Neuroscience 2011, Dec 7; 31 (49); 17821.

[114] Cramer Bornemann, Michel A, Mahowald MW. Sleep forensics. In: Principles and Practice of Sleep Medicine. St. Louis: Saunders, Elsivier; 2011. p. 725-33.

[115] Ohayon MM, Mahowald MW, Leger D. Are confusional arousals pathological? Neurology 2014, Aug 26; 83 (9); 834-41.

Section 3

Sleep Apnoea

Chapter 4

Obstructive Sleep Apnea Syndrome in Childhood

Leila A. Azevedo, Heidi H. Sander,
Wilma T. Anselmo-Lima and Fabiana C.P. Valera

Additional information is available at the end of the chapter

http://dx.doi.org/10.5772/57885

1. Introduction

Obstructive Sleep Apnea Syndrome (OSAS) is a condition characterized by intermittent partial or total obstruction of the upper airways during sleep. The events of upper airway obstruction are associated with repetitive episodes of hypoxemia and microarousals, usually followed by autonomic activation. As a consequence, OSAS is related to sleep fragmentation, excessive daytime sleepiness and its consequences, cognitive and behavioural changes, and an increased risk of cardiovascular and cerebrovascular diseases.[1]

In childhood, OSAS is characterized by both intermittent obstruction and by prolonged periods of partial resistance/obstruction of the airways.[1] Methodological differences in diagnosing this disease have led to variable reports of prevalence, with the strongest evidence indicating a prevalence of 1 to 5%.2 The disease occurs in all childhood age ranges from the neonatal period to adolescence, being more common among preschoolers.

In the childhood age range, OSAS is more frequently associated with tonsil and adenoid hypertrophy and with other conditions including obesity, allergic rhinitis, craniofacial malformations, neuromuscular diseases, and genetic and metabolic syndromes.

Important clinical outcomes of the condition such as delayed growth and hyperactive behavior have been well established. [1]

2. Clinical aspects

Clinical Signs and Symptoms: The clinical signs and symptoms are mainly characterized by snoring, difficult breathing during sleep, nighttime breathing pauses, agitated sleep, and hyperactive behavior.

Snoring is present in the great majority of children, but may not be observed in infants or children with muscle weakness. Paradoxical breathing is frequently present due to a more complying thoracic cage in childhood.1

Different ventilatory patterns may characterize Sleep Disordered Breathing (SDB) in childhood, with the predominance or exclusive presence of each one in each child: [1]

1. Cyclic apneas, as observed in adults, with snoring associated with intermittent breathing pauses followed by noisy inspiraton and movements/microarousals.

2. Obstructive hypoventilation, with continuous snoring, without frequent pauses or microarousals. This pattern occurs in younger children and consists of prolonged periods of *partial* airway obstruction associated with hypercapnia or hypoxemia, or both.

3. A pattern similar to that known in adults as Upper Airway Resistance Syndrome, with snoring and intermittent periods of greater ventilatory effort associated with microarousals, with no changes in flow compatible with apnea or hypopnea.

In childhood, respiratory events may occur without being associated with microarousals, especially in younger children, due to the high arousal threshold. In addition, these events occur more during REM sleep, when the child is especially predisposed not to wake, and are rare during slow-wave sleep. [1] Typically, there is greater preservation of sleep architecture than in adults. For this purpose, the main pattern of sleep architecture change is the increase of slow-wave sleep and a reduction of REM sleep duration. [3, 4]

Snoring is usually reported by the caregivers, whereas breathing pauses may not be perceived. Or, conversely, the parents may report the observation of nighttime breathing pauses in children, with these events being of the central type – or even obstructive – but of an insufficient number to characterize OSAS. Thus, anamnesis alone is insufficient to exclude or diagnose sleep apnea in children who snore. [5, 6, 7, 8, 9]

In addition to snoring and breathing pauses, other signs observed are agitated sleep, night sweats, preferential decubitus with cervical hyperextension, and enuresis. Episodes of parasomnia and sleep bruxism may be more frequent. Morning headache, difficulty in getting up in the morning and excessive daytime sleepiness may occur, especially among older children. Excessive sleepiness is usually absent in younger children, who more commonly show daytime agitation.

Since tonsil and adenoid hypertrophy is the main cause underlying OSAS in the childhood age range, related clinical aspects may be present, such as mouth breathing syndrome and its orthodontic and craniofacial complications such as crossbite, high-arched palate, and long face syndrome with practically constant open mouth (figure 1); dysphagia and odynophagia; repeated upper airway infections; hearing loss; gastroesophageal reflux disease. So far, the degree of tonsil and adenoid hypertrophy has not been documented to predict the presence of OSAS in children who snore and are mouth breathers. [10, 11] Methodological aspects may be involved, in addition to the fact that other factors contribute to the presence or absence of OSAS, such as particularities of the neural control of ventilation in each child.

In younger children, OSAS may be related to difficulty in gaining weight, particularly when associated with genetic syndromes. In older children, obesity may be present. Regardless of their weight status, children may develop weight gain after treatment of OSAS, not infrequently increasing their food intake after improvement of olfaction, of dysphagia and of odynophagia induced by adenotonsillectomy. 1

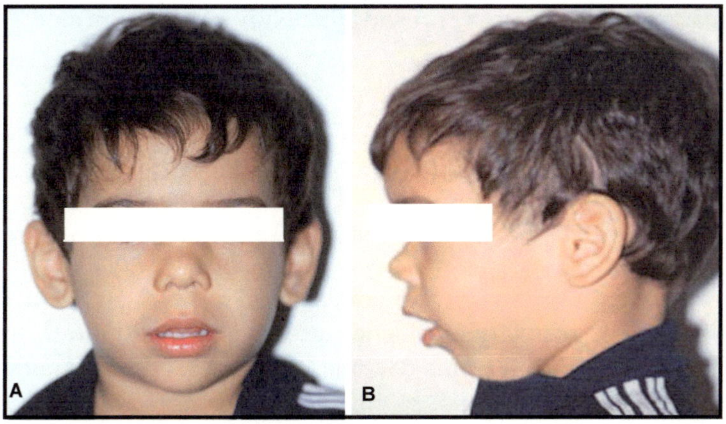

Figure 1. Typical face in mouth breathing children. **(A)** frontal; **(B)** lateral view.

Some of the clinical outcomes of this syndrome in childhood have been well established, whereas others are still under investigation. The complaint of school difficulty is relatively frequent and most studies have established an association between childhood OSAS and cognitive deficit. However, the correlation between the severity of the breathing disorder and the degree of neuropsychological impairment is still controversial due to methodological differences and to the lack of control of other relevant clinical variables such as obesity, in addition to environmental and social variables. More studies are still needed to determine the cognitive subdomains that are more affected, their relationship with hypoxemia and sleep fragmentation, and their evolution after the treatment of OSAS.[2]

From a behavioral viewpoint, hyperactive behavior is the most common abnormality. Children tend to show a worse performance in tests of sustained attention and executive functions [12, 13] and may or may not fulfill the formal criteria of Attention Deficit Hyperactivity Disorder (ADHD). In addition, children with ADHD have a higher prevalence of SDB than controls.[14, 15, 16] Aggressiveness, difficulty in social relations, and mood changes are other behaviors reported.

Excessive daytime sleepiness may be present in some children, although few studies have correlated polysomnography (PSG) parameters with objective sleepiness parameters.[2]

Some studies have demonstrated behavioral and cognitive improvement after the treatment of apnea in children, whereas others have detected persistence of the previous impairment. [2] Well-designed studies are still needed, with the control of confounding variables such as family and social environment, educational level, time of disease evolution, and the presence of other sleep disorders.

Regarding the cardiovascular outcomes, despite the scarcity of well-designed studies, there is evidence indicating increased arterial pressure and repercussions on both the right and left ventricles. Arterial hypertension, pulmonary hypertension and *cor pulmonale* may occur in children with more severe disorder. There is a lack of well- controlled studies also regarding inflammatory markers, with C-reactive protein apparently increasing in more serious cases. [2]

3. Diagnosis

Ideally, the presence of OSAS should be investigated in all children with complaints of snoring and agitated sleep. However, the predictive value of the clinical history alone is low, with PSG being considered to be the gold standard for diagnosis. [17] Alternative methods of diagnostic complementation such as oximetry, evaluation of cardiovascular parameters, ambulatory evaluation of ventilatory parameters, and daytime PSG have not been recommended to define the diagnosis thus far, as they may not be sufficient when negative. Ideally, children with negative results should be referred to whole night PSG study. [2]

A	Report of snoring or of increased breathing effort, or both during sleep
B.	The caregiver or the child reports at least ONE of the signs/symptoms below: 1. presence of a paradoxical breathing pattern during inspiration 2. arousal associated with movements 3. diaphoresis 4. cervical hyperextension during sleep 5. excessive daytime sleepiness, hyperactivity or aggressive behavior 6. reduced growth rate 7. morning headache 8. secondary nighttime enuresis
C.	PSG presents obstructive AHI ≥ 1/hour
D.	PSG presents items 1 or 2 below: 1. At least ONE of the events below: 1.1. increased arousals related to increased breathing effort; 1.2. fall in oxygen saturation associated with obstructive breathing events; 1.3. hypercapnia during sleep; 1.4. marked negative oscillation in esophageal pressure 2. Periods of hypercapnia or desaturation, or both, during sleep, associated with snoring, paradoxical breathing and at least one of the events below: 2.1. frequent arousals; 2.2. marked negative oscillation of esophageal pressure

Table 1. Diagnosis of OSAS in Childhood and Adolescence

According to the criteria of the International Classification of Sleep Disorders [1], the diagnosis is based on clinical and PSG criteria (Table 1). From a clinical viewpoint, there must be the complaint of snoring and/or difficult breathing during the night, associated with at least one of the following signs and symptoms: paradoxical breathing, agitated sleep, nocturnal sudoresis, cervical hyperextension, excessive daytime sleepness, hyperactivity or aggressive behavior, morning headache, and secondary enuresis.

From a polysomnographic viewpoint, an Apnea + Hypopnea Index (AHI) ≥ 1/hour should be present in association with sleep fragmentation, desaturation episodes, hypercapnia, or negative oscillations of esophageal pressure.

4. Clinical and complementary evaluation

4.1. Clinical evaluation and physical examination: Anterior rhinoscopy and endoscopy

The systematized measurement of cervical circumference routinely used for adults has not been standardized for children and therefore it is not routinely used in most services.

The otorhinolaryngology exam is always focused on the search of obstructive causes in the airways, from the nasal fossae to the regions of the hypopharynx and larynx. Bone changes such as micrognathia and deformity of the skull base (present, for example in individuals with Down Syndrome) should always be remembered. Complementary flexible nasofibroscopy is desirable, as it permits a precise evaluation up to the larynx region. The main causes of respiratory obstruction are:

Choanal Atresia: this is a congenital malformation that leads to nasal obstruction, nasal secretion and, when bilateral, respiratory stress breathing at birth. The diagnosis can be made by CT scan and nasal endoscopy (Figure 2).

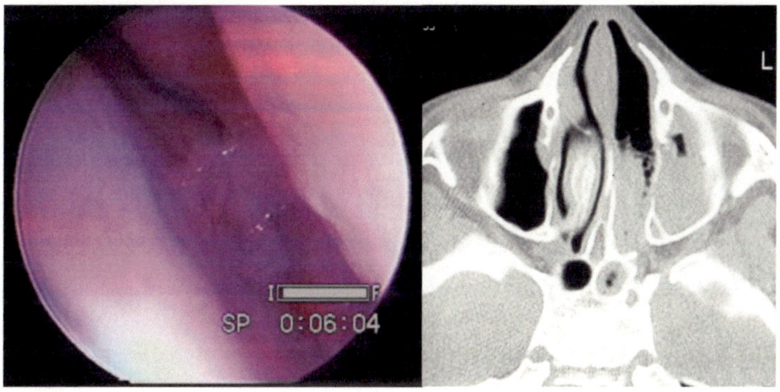

Figure 2. Choanal Atresia. **(A)** Endoscopic view: posterior nasal fossa, left side, with impermeable choana; **(B)** Axial CT scan, showing the choanal atresia at the left side.

Adenotonsillar hypertrophy: the complaints reported by the mother usually starts when the child is already older than two years, although they may also start earlier. Depending on the severity of the case, the child has nighttime apnea which considerably frightens the parents, who are unable to sleep. Diagnosis of palatine tonsils hypertrophy is clinical (Figure 3), while adenoid hypertrophy, in most cases, the diagnosis is confirmed by simple lateral radiography or nasofibroscopy (Figure 4). It should be pointed out that Valera et al.[18], in 2005, in a retrospective study based on the analysis of clinical data in the medical records of 267 children, did not observe a correlation between the degree of adenotonsillary hypertrophy and the severity of OSAS. These data were later confirmed by Nolan and Brietzke (2011) [10], who concluded that the association between tonsil grading and OSAS severity should be considered at best weak.

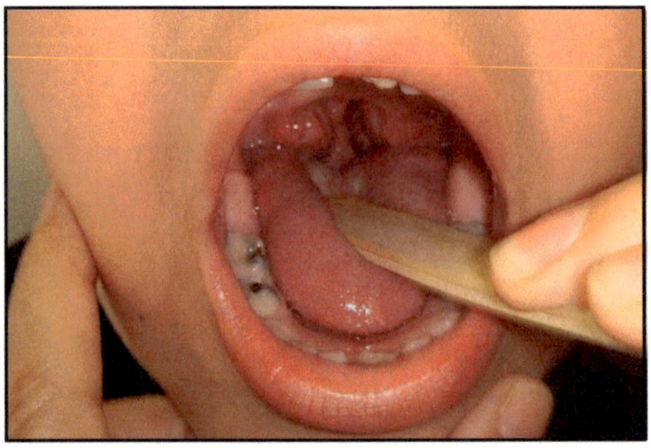

Figure 3. Grade IV palatine tonsils

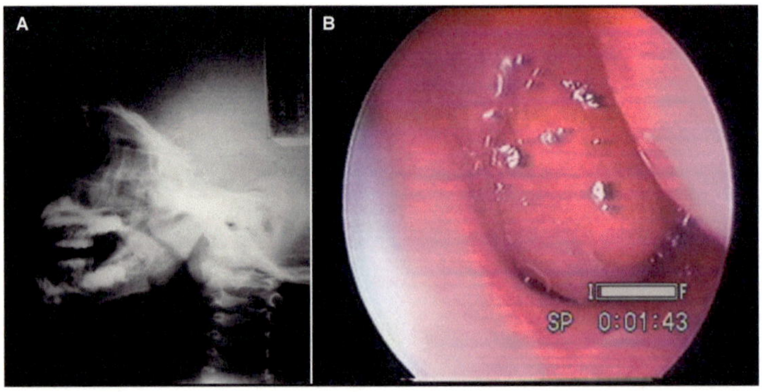

Figure 4. Adenoid hypertrophy. **(A)** Lateral X-Ray; **(B)** Endoscopic view, with important obstruction in nasopharynx due to adenoid hypertrophy.

Allergic rhinitis: children with allergic rhinitis who are not properly treated may present severe nasal obstruction because the hypertrophic nasal turbinates prevent the airflow.

Anatomical variations of the nasal turbinates: the most common of them is the Bollosa turbinate, when the middle turbinate is pneumatized. This variation may be only a endoscopic/ radiographic finding, but it may be also related to nasal obstruction and repeated rhinosinusitis. The diagnostic suspicion based on nasofibroscopy is confirmed by CT scan (Figure 5).

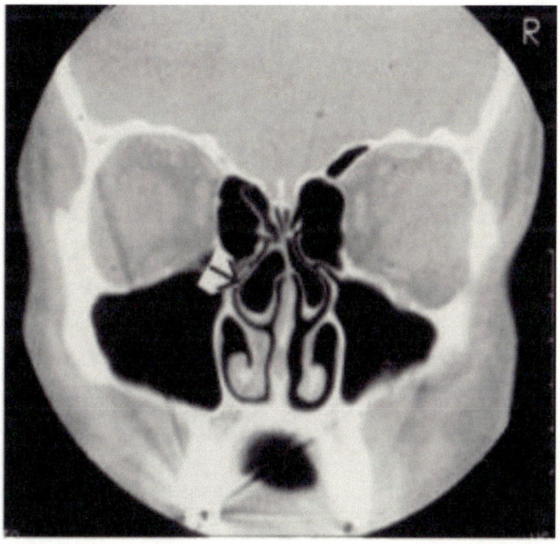

Figure 5. Cororal CT scan, showing bilateral concha bollosa

Septal deformities: important deviations of the septal wall can also induce mouth breathing and OSAS in children (Figure 6).

Nasal tumors: benign or malignant tumors in the nasal fossae of children may provoke unilateral or bilateral nasal obstruction and should be promptly diagnosed (Figures 7 to 9).

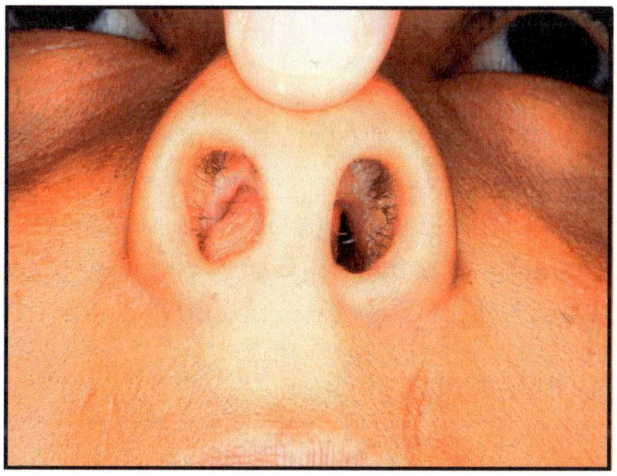

Figure 6. Anterior septal deviation.

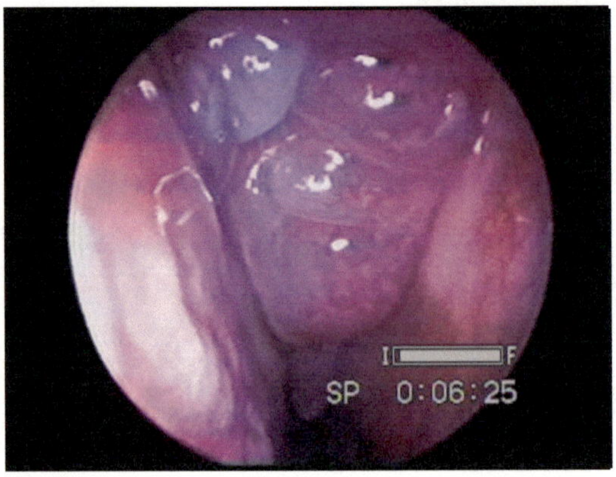

Figure 7. Endoscopic view: Nasal polyps.

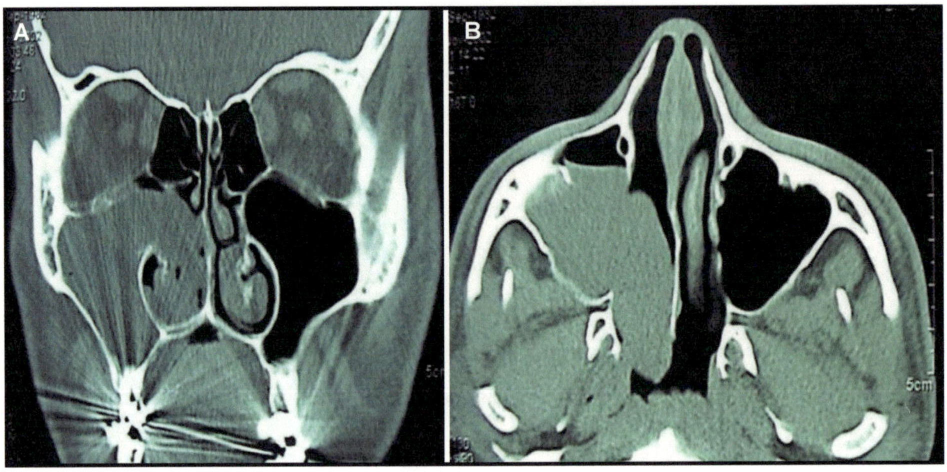

Figure 8. Anthrochoanal polyp **(A)** Coronal CT scan; **(B)** Axial CT scan.

Flexible nasal fibroscopy should reach the region of the larynx, also for the evaluation of changes in soft tissues such as macroglossia and of laryngeal diseases such as laryngomalacia (Figure 10). The procedure permits the diagnosis of hypotonia of the dilators of the lower airways present in children with neuromuscular abnormalities (hypotonic muscular dystrophies and cerebral palsy causing lack of coordination).

Some authors[19] recommend the use of anterior rhinomanometry, which measures nasal resistance in order to diagnose severe apnea in children. According to them, the nasal resistance of children is significantly reduced with age and increases in the presence of edema of the nasal fossae induced by adenoid enlargement. However, this exam is not routinely performed in these children.

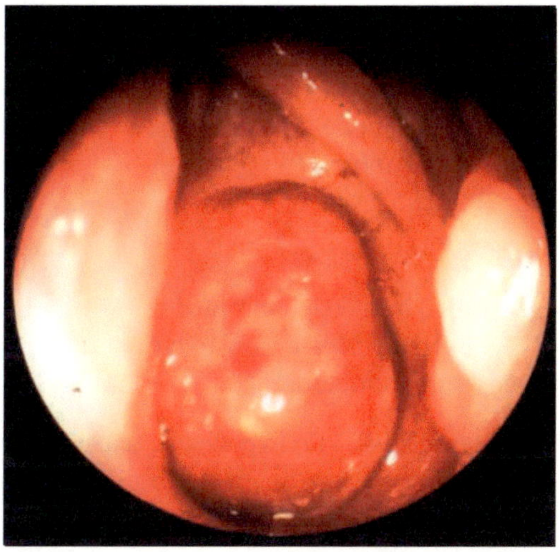

Figure 9. Endoscopic view of nasopharynx: nasopharyngeal tumor diagnosed as naso lymphoma.

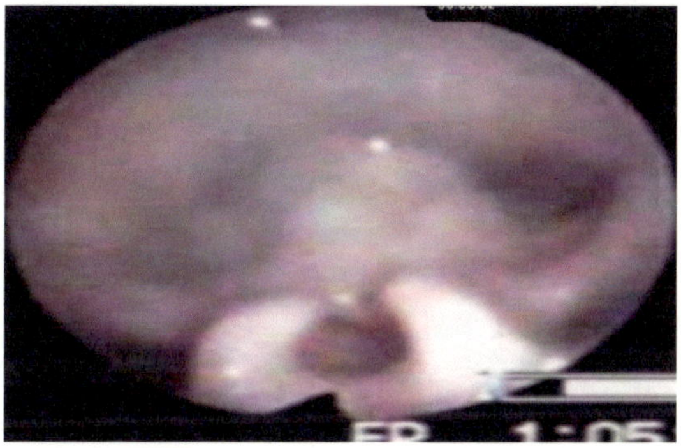

Figure 10. Endoscopic view of laryngomalacia. Reduncdant arythenoyd tissue, obstructing laryngeal glottis.

4.2. Cephalometry

In view of the interaction between craniofacial changes and SDB in children, cephalometry is considered to be a useful exam for these patients. [20] The exam consists of radiography of the face in a systematic manner, so that the data for one patient can be compared to a data bank of normal values.

However, its routine use for the evaluation of patients with OSAS is still questioned by the major consensuses. [21] According to these consensuses, clinical evaluation can identify the main craniofacial changes when they are more exuberant and this should determine whether the patient needs cephalometry as an additional exam. Cephalometry, however, is essential for the indication of surgery in patients with craniofacial anaomalies.

All professionals who deal with children should be aware these as the main causes of OSAS in children and refer these patients to a specialist who will detect them and treat them correctly as soon as possible. Permitting the child to breathe through the nose before five years of age prevents the installation of changes of bone development and of facial muscles and will favor growth with the desired orofacial harmony.

4.3. Polysomnography

Nocturnal polysomnography (PSG) in a sleep laboratory is considered to be the gold standard for the evaluation of SDB since it provides an objective and quantitative evaluation of the respiratory and sleep architecture parameters [17].

Despite the scarcity of sleep laboratories with experience in treating children, diagnostic PSG recording in childhood can be acquired with few technical variations compared to adult examination, with the most important differential probably being the incorporation of capnography. The interpretation of the recording should be adapted to the childhood age range and the recommendation is to acquire and analyze the data according to the pediatric criteria of the sleep staging manual of the American Academy of Sleep Medicine (AASM) [22]. These criteria should be applied for children and adolescents up to 18 years of age, although, in selected cases, adult criteria can be applied to individuals older than 13 years.

Apneas should be identified by recording oronasal airflow with a thermistor, and hypopneas should be identified with pressure transducers using a nasal pressure tube [22].

The main events identified are:

1. Obstructive apnea: A reduction of basal air flow of 90% or more for at least two breathing cycles, accompanied by breathing effort.

2. Mixed apnea: A reduction of basal air flow of 90% or more for at least two breathing cycles, with breathing effort present only during one period of absence of airflow.

3. Central apnea: A reduction of basal air flow of 90% or more in the absence of breathing effort. Central apneas lasting more than 20 seconds and central apneas with a duration of two respiratory cycles accompanied by desaturation $\geq 3\%$ or arousal are computed. For children younger than 1 year, only central apneas associated with a reduction of heart rate of less than 50 bpm for at least 5 seconds, or less than 60 bpm for at least 15 seconds are considered.

4. Hypopnea: Reduction of at least 30% of the amplitude of the pressure tube signal for two respiratory cycles accompanied by desaturation of $\geq 3\%$ or arousal. When breathing effort is maintained, obstructive hypopnea is considered to be present [2].

In children, for the diagnosis and classification of SDB, no effect of the first night responsible for erroneous stratification of the disease was observed. The night-to-night variation of AHI in consecutive PSG or PSG performed at intervals of up to 50 days does not seem to be significant in children aged 2 to 17 years [23, 24, 25, 26, 27, 28]. In this respect, the recording of one night is usually adequate for the diagnostic evaluation of SDB.

Few studies have specifically assessed the accuracy of PSG for the diagnosis of OSAS in children. The fragility of the correlation between PSG parameters and the remaining aspects of the disease, such as the clinical itself does not necessarily indicate poor validation of PSG, since these aspects may not have the reliability or stability needed to represent a useful comparative measurement. Also, test-test tests after intervention studies have provided moderate to strong evidence of the validity of PSG for the characterization of childhood SDB. Also, reliability and reproducibility tests provide good to excellent support for the use of PSG in the evaluation of ventilatory parameters in infants and children. [17, 28]

In summary, the PSG exam in children is probably useful, valid and reproducible and, when interpreted in the light of clinical data, it represents the gold standard for the diagnosis of SDB also in the childhood age range.

5. Treatment

Pharmacological Treatment. Since the major cause of OSAS in children is adenotonsillary hypertrophy [22], the initial treatment should approach these structures.

For children with adenoid hypertrophy alone, the intial treatment could be the use of topical nasal corticosteroids. The use of mometasone furoate, for example, has been effective in reducing the dimensions of the adenoids and in improving the obstructive symptoms. [29, 30, 31] There is no evidence about treatment with Montelucast alone.

Adenotonsillectomy should be considered in cases in which there is association with hypertrophy of the palatine tonsils and in cases that did not respond adequately to clinical treatment.

Adenotonsillectomy. Adenotonsillectomy is considered to be the main treatment of OSAS in childhood. [2, 32] This is a procedure with a high benefit/risk ratio[2], since it is highly efficient and presents a low prevalence of complications. Major complications are bleeding, infection, anesthetic complications, respiratory decompensation, velopharyngeal incompetence, subglottic stenosis and, rarely, death.

Despite the low postoperative risks in general, there is a pediatric population that is especially susceptible to complications: patients younger than 3 years, with severe OSAS, with cardiac complications, difficulty in gaining weight, important craniofacial changes, genetic syndromes, and neuromuscular diseases. All of these children should be submitted to adenotonsillectomy in a tertiary hospital, where prompt admission to the pediatric ICU would be possible.[33] In addition, the American Academy of Otolaryngology-Head and Neck Surgery recommends that children with AHI ≥ 10/h and/or Nadir of $SATO_2$< 80% be admitted for observation after adenotonsillectomy. [34]

Partial tonsillectomy is not indicated since it may cause greater perioperative bleeding, maintenance of repeated infections and recurrence of obstruction due to new tissue growth. [2]

Relative contraindications of adenotonsillectomy for OSAS are: a small tonsil and adenoid size, acute infection of the upper airways, untreated hemorrhagic disease, or other clinical conditions that cause patient instability for the surgical procedure.

Adenotonsillectomy has proved to reduce AHI significantly when compared to preoperative values. [32, 35, 36, 37] The rates of cure obtained with adenotonsillectomy vary according to the definition of OSAS used, to the definition of cure criteria and to sample differences, such as the proportion of obese children among the subjects operated. For AHI ≥ 1/h the rates of OSAS persistence after adenotonsillectomy vary from 19 to 73%. Consistent risk factors for residual OSAS reported in the literature are obesity and severity of preoperative OSAS. The absence of postoperative snoring represents a good parameter for reevaluation, although it is not 100% specific. Thus, PSG should be performed after surgery in children at risk for residual disease.

In addition to improving AHI, adenotonsillectomy is associated with an improvement of the quality of life, of behavior, of cognitive function, and of oral motricity. [38, 39, 4, 41] Another benefit, mainly observed in children of preschool age, is the reversal of some craniofacial changes: in some studies, adenotonsillectomy led to greater transverse palatal growth, to compensation of anterior crossbite and to a reduction of mandibular inclination.[42, 43, 44, 45, 46, 47]

Rapid maxillary expansion. Rapid maxillary expansion (RME) is an orthodontic procedure for the enlargement of the transverse diameter of the hard palate by the redimension of the palatine suture, which may be an alternative for children with maxillary constriction and malocclusion.

RME is only indicated when the children present concomitant maxillary atresia, preferably associated with unilateral or bilateral crossbite and when the maxillary symphysis has not yet undergone fusion. In some studies conducted by the Stanford group, [48, 49, 50] RME was associated with a significant improvement of apnea indiceses and with an improved quality of life.

Despite this proven improvement of PSG indices, there still is some controversy about the effect of RME on the enlargement of nasal dimensions: while some studies have demonstrated an increased volume and a reduced nasal resistance, [51, 52, 53, 54] others have not been able to demonstrate this effect.[55, 56, 57] The same conflict occurs regarding enlargement of the pharynx: while Iwasaki et al.[58] observed an increased pharyngeal volume by cone-beam tomography, Ribeiro et al.[59] and Langer et al.[60] detected no effect of RME on nasopharyngeal volume.

Thus, the effect of RME on childhood OSAS needs to be better elucidated for a better understanding of the mechanism responsible for this clinical improvement and for the confirmation of its real benefit.

Positive Pressure Therapy. Despite the treatments described above, some degree of residual OSAS persists in many children, who continue to experience apnea even after optimized clinical/surgical treatment. [32, 61] This persistence is mainly observed in older children, in children with associated obesity and asthma, and in children with more severe apnea during the preopeative period. [32, 36] In cases of residual OSAS in children with craniofacial anomalies, skeletal treatment (clinical, with orthodontic braces or surgical) can optimize the improvement and, in many cases, reverse the persistence of OSAS. However, the treatment most indicated for cases of moderate to severe residual OSAS is continuous positive airway pressure (CPAP). [2]

CPAP is used in general in children with persistent moderate to severe disease after surgical correction, especially obese children, children with craniofacial anomalies or children with contraindication of surgery. Treatment with CPAP is associated with improvement of clinical symptoms and of PSG parameters.

Despite a significant improvement in respiratory parameters and in quality of life, a problem with the use of CPAP in children in the rate of adhesion: according to Marcus et al, [62] one third of the children abandon the use of the device by six months after its indication. Thus, the success of therapy depends on greater efforts for obtaining adequate nasal or oronasal interfaces, education, support and parental counseling.

Bilevel positive airway pressure (BiPAP) therapy is indicated for children with comorbidities that lead to the absence or insufficiency of the ventilatory drive, such as sequelae of cardiorespiratory arrest and Moebius Syndrome, or hypoventilation secondary to neuromuscular diseases or chest wall deformities.

Special Conditions. Children with craniofacial abnormalities, genetic syndromes, sequelae of a hypoxic-ischemic insult and neuromuscular diseases should receive individualized treatment that might contemplate adenotonsillectomy, specific treatment of the base disease, when present, procedures for facial deformities such as mandibular distraction, and therapy with positive pressure. Tracheostomy is indicated when CPAP/BIiPAP treatment is impossible or fails in children with very severe OSAS, or may be performed transitorily during the perioperative period in airway surgeries in children at risk for respiratory insufficiency.

6. Future research

The described flow diagram for the therapeutic approach to OSAS is not so simple, with many children who do not present the principal risk factors continuing to have OSAS after surgery, while others continue to have mild symptoms of low clinical importance for their parents.

At present, these children pose the greatest difficulty of conduct:

- Should partial polysonographic improvement be treated even when the child continues to be asymptomatic?
- If so, which treatment should be indicated?
- May mild residual OSAS predispose this child to becoming an adult with OSAS?

- All of these questions, although occasionally answered, should be further explored in the near future so that more appropriate therapeutic conducts can be offered to the pediatric population.

Author details

Leila A. Azevedo, Heidi H. Sander, Wilma T. Anselmo-Lima and Fabiana C.P. Valera

Medical School of Ribeirão Preto - University of São Paulo, Brazil

References

[1] American Academy of Sleep Medicine. International classification of sleep disorders, 2^{end}.: Diagnostic and coding manual. Westchester, Illinois: American Academy of Sleep Medicine, 2005.

[2] Marcus CL, Brooks LJ, Ward SD et al. Diagnosis and Manegement of Childhood Obstructive Sleep Apnea Syndrome. *Pediatrics* 2012;(130):714-55.

[3] Tauman R, O'Brien LM, Holbrook CR et al. Sleep pressure score: a new index of sleep disruption in snoring children. *Sleep* 2004;27(2):274-8.

[4] Gozal D, Wang M, Pope DW. Objective sleepiness measures in pediatric obstructive sleep apnea. Pediatrics 2001;(108):693-7.

[5] Carrol JL, McColley SA, Marcus CL. Inability of clinical history to distinguish primary snoring from obstructive sleep apnea syndrome in children. *Chest* 1995;(108): 610-618.

[6] Chan CH, Ng DK. Apnea-hypopnea index as the outcome variable in multiple linear regression analysis: statistical issues. *Pediat Pulmonol* 2007;42(8):711-5.

[7] Gozal D, Gozal LK. New approaches to the diagnosis of sleep-disordered breathing in children. *Sleep Medicine* 2010;(11):708-713.

[8] Kaditis A, Gozal LK, Gozal D et al. Algorithm for the diagnosis and treatment of pedicatric OSA: A proposal of two pediatric sleep centers. *Sleep Medicine* 2012;13:217-227.

[9] Moréa EE, Isemb FS, Zumela PH et al. Efectividad clínica y polisomnográfica de la adenamigdalectomía en el tratamento de los transtornos respiratórios del sueño en los ninõs. *Acta Otorrinolaringol Esp* 2008;59(7):325-33.

[10] Nolan J, Brietzke, S.E. Systematic Review of Pediatric Tonsil Size and Polysomnogram-Measured Obstructive Sleep Apnea Severity. *Otolaryngology-Head and Neck Surgery* 2011;144: 844-850.

[11] Tagaya et al. Relationship between adenoid size and severity of obstructive sleep apnea in preschool children. *International Journal of Pediatric Otorhinolaryngology* 2012;76:1827–1830.

[12] O'Brien LM, Mervis CB, Holbrook CR et al: Neurobehavioral correlates of sleep-disordered breathing in children. *J Sleep Res* 2004; 13:165.

[13] Lewin DS, Rosen RC, England SJ, Dahl R.: Preliminary evidence of behavioral and cognitive sequelae of obstructive sleep apnea in children. *J Sleep Res* 2002; 3:5.

[14] Chervin RD, Dillon JE, Bassetti C et al: Sleep-disordered breathing and behavior in three risk groups: preliminary findings from parental reports. *Childs Nerv Syst* 1993;9:452.

[15] Chervin RD, Archbold KH, Dillon JE et al: Inattention, hyperactivity, and symptoms of sleep-disordered breathing. *Pediatrics* 2002; 109:449.

[16] Chervin RD, Ruzicka DL, Archbold KH, Dillon JE: Snoring predicts hyperactivity four years later. *Sleep* 2005; 28:885.

[17] Wise MS et al. Executive summary of respiratory indications for polysomnography in children: an evidence–based review. *Sleep*, 2011; 34(3):389-398.

[18] Valera FCP, Avelino MAG, Pettermann MB, et al. OSAS in children: correlation between endoscopic and polysomnographic findings. *Otolaryngol Head Neck Surg.* 2005;132:268-72.

[19] Rizzi M, Onorato J, Andreoli A et al. Nasal resistances are useful in identifying children with severe obstructive sleep apnea before polysomnography. *International Journal of Pediatric Otorhinolaryngology* 2002 (65): 7–13.

[20] Avrahami E, Englender M. Relation between CT axial cross-sectional area of the oropharynx and obstructive sleep apnea syndrome in adults. *Am J Neuro-radiol.* 1995; 16:135-40.

[21] Marcus CL et al. Pathophysiology of childhood obstructive sleep apnea: current concepts. *Respiration Physiology* 2000;119:143–154.

[22] The American Academy of Sleep Medicine Manual for the Scoring of Sleep and Associated Events, version 2.0, 2012. http://www.aasmnet.org/scoringmanual/htlm.

[23] Katz ES et al. Night-to-night variability of polysomnography in children with suspected obstructive sleep apnea. *The Journal of Pediatrics*, 2002; 140:589-594.

[24] Li AM et al. Is a 2-night polysomnographic study necessary in childhood sleep-related disordered breathing?. *Chest*, 2004; 126:1467-1472.

[25] Verhulst SL et al. First night effect for polysomnography data in children and adolescents with suspected sleep disordered breathing. *Arch Dis Child*, 2006; 91: 233-237.

[26] Scholle S et al. First night effect in children and adolescents undergoing polysomnogrqaphy for sleep-disordered breathing. *Clinical Neurophysiology*, 2003; 114: 2138-2145.

[27] Goodwin JL et al. Feasibility of using unattended polysomnography in children for research – report of the Tucson Children's Assessment of Sleep Apnea Study (TuCASA). *Sleep*, 2001; 24(8): 937-944.

[28] Wise MS et al. Respiratory indications for polysomnography in children: an evidence-based review. *Sleep*, 2011; 34(3): 398A-398AW.

[29] Zhang L, Mendoza-Sassi RA, César JA et al. Intranasal corticosteroids for nasal airway obstruction in children with moderate to severe adenoidal hypertrophy. *Cochrane Database Syst Rev*. 2008; 16(3): CD006286.

[30] Chadha NK, Zhang L, Mendoza-Sassi RA, César JA et al. Using nasal steroids to treat nasal obstruction caused by adenoid hypertrophy: does it work? *Otolaryngol Head Neck Surg*. 2009; 140(2): 139-47.

[31] Rezende RN, Silveira F, Barbosa AP et al. Objective reduction in adenoid tissue after mometasone furoate treatment. *Int J Pediatr Otorhinolaryngol*. 2012; 76: 829-31.

[32] Bhattacharjee R, Gozal KL, Spruyt K et al. Adenotonsillectomy outcomes in treatment of obstructive sleep apnea in children. *Am J Respir Crit Care Med*. 2010; 182: 676-83.

[33] Schwengel DA, Sterni LM, Tunkel D et al. Perioperative management of children with obstructive sleep apnea. *Anesth Analg* 2009;109:60-75.

[34] Roland OS, Rosenfeld RM, Brooks LJ et al. American Academy of Otolalyngology-Head and Neck Surgery Foundation. Clinical practice guideline: Polysomnography for sleep-disordered breathing prior to tonsillectomy in children. *Otolaryngol Head Neck Surg*. 2001;145(suppl 1):S1-S15.

[35] Brietzke SE. Gallangher D. The effectiveness of tonsillectomy and adenoidectomy in the treatment of pediatric obstructive sleep apnea/ hypopnea syndrome: a meta-analysis. *Otolaryngol Head Neck Surg*. 2006; 134: 979-84.

[36] Tauman R, Gulliver TE, Krishna J, Montomery-Downs HE, O'Brien LM, Ivanenko A, et al. Persistence of obstructive sleep apnea syndrome in children after adenotonillectomy. *J Pediatr*. 2006; 149: 803-8.

[37] Friedman M, Wilson M, Lin HC, Chang HW. Uptated systematic review of tonsillectomy and adenoidectomy for treatment of pediatric obstructive sleep apnea/ hypopnea syndrome. *Otolaryngol Head Neck Surg*. 2009; 140: 800-8.

[38] Ericsson E, Ledin T, Hultcrantz E. Long-term improvement of quality of life as a resullt of tonsillotomy (with radiofrequency technique) and tonsillectomy in youths. *Laryngoscope.* 2007; 117(7): 1272-9.

[39] Baldassari CM, Mitchell RB, Schubert C, Rudnick EF. Pediatric obstructive sleep apnea and quality of life: a meta-analysis. *Otolaryngol Head Neck Surg.* 2008; 138: 265-73.

[40] De la Chaux R, Klemens C, Patscheider M, Reichel O, Dreher A. Tonsillotomy in the treatment of obstructive sleep apnea synfrome in children: polysomnographic results. *Int J Pediatr Otorhinolaryngol.* 2008 72: 1411-7.

[41] Valera FCP, Trawitzki LVV, Anselmo-Lima WT. Myofunctional evaluation after surgery for tonsils hypertrophy and its correlation to breathing pattern: a 2-year-follow up. *Int J Pediatr Otorhinolaryngol.* 2006; 70: 221-5.

[42] Vieira BB, Sanguino ACM, Mattar SE, Itikawa CE, Anselmo-Lima WT, Valera FCP, Matsumoto MAN. Influence of adenotonsillectomy on hard palate dimensions. *Int J Pediatr Otorhinolaryngol.* 2012; 76(8): 1140-4.

[43] Mattar SE, Valera FCP, Faria G, Matsumoto MAN, Anselmo-Lima WT. Changes in facial morphology after adenotonsillectomy in mouth-breathing children. *Int J Peadiatr Dent.* 2011; 21(5): 389-96.

[44] Mattar SE, Matsumoto MAN, Valera FCP, Anselmo-Lima WT, Faria G. The effect of adenoidectomy or adenotonsillectomy on occlusal features in mouth-breathing preschoolers. *Pediatr Dent.* 2012; 34(2): 108-12.

[45] Mahony D, Karsten A, Linder-Aronson S. Effects of adenoidectomy and changed mode of breathing on incisor and molar dentoalveolar heights and anterior face heights. *Aust Orthod J.* 2004; 20(2): 93-8.

[46] Peltomäki T. The effect of mode of breathing on craniofacial growth-revisited. *Eur J Orthod.* 2007; 29(5): 426-9.

[47] Souki BQ, Pimenta GB, Franco LP, Becker HM, Pinto JA. Changes in vertical dentofacial morphology after adenotonsillectomy during deciduous and mixed dentitions mouth breathing children – 1 year follow-up study. *Int J Pediatr Otorhinolaryngol.* 2010; 74(6): 626-32.

[48] Villa MP, Malagola C, Pagani J, Montesano M, Rizzoli A, Guilleminault C, et al. Rapid maxillary expansion in children with obstructive sleep apnea syndrome: 12-month follow-up. *Sleep Med.* 2007; 8: 128.

[49] Guilleminault C, Quo S, Huynh NT, Li K. Orthodontic expansion treatment and adenotonsillectomy in the treatment of obstructive sleep apnea in prepubertal children. *Sleep.* 2008; 31: 953-7.

[50] Guilleminault C, Monteyrol PJ, Huynh NT, Pirelli P, Quo S, Li K. Adeno-tonsillectomy and rapid maxillary distraction in pre-pubertal children, a pilot study. *Sleep Breath.* 2011; 15: 173-7.

[51] De Felipe NL, Bhushan N, Da Silveira AC, Viana G, Smith B. Long-term effect of orthodontic therapy on the maxillary dental arch and nasal cavity. *Am J Orthod Dentofacial Orthop.* 2009; 136(4): 490.e1-8.

[52] Söküсü O, Doruk C, Uysal OI. Comparison of the effects of RME and fan-type RME on nasal airway by using acoustic rhinometry. *Angle Orthod. 2010*; 80(5): 870-5.

[53] Baratieri C, Alves M Jr, de Souza MM, de Souza Araújo MT, Maia LC. Does rapid maxillary exapansion have long-term effects on airway dimensions and breathing? *Am J Orthod Dentofacial Orthop.* 2011; 140(2): 146-56.

[54] Torre H, Alarcón JA. Changes in nasal air flow and should grades after rapid maxillary expansion in oral breathing children. *Mod Oral Patol Oral Cir Bucal.* 2012; 17(5): e865-70.

[55] Enoki C, Valera FCP, Lessa FCR, Elias AM, Matsumoto MAN, Anselmo-Lima WT. Effects of rapid maxillary expansion on the dimensiono f the nasal cavity and on nasal air resistance. *Int J Ped Otorhinolaryngol* 2006; 70: 1225-30.

[56] Matsumoto MAN, Itikawa CE, Valera FCP, Faria G, Anselmo-Lima WT. Long-term effects of rapid maxillary expansion on nasal área and nasal airway resistance. *Am J Rhinol Allergy* 2010; 24: 161-5.

[57] Johnson BM, McNamara JA, Bandeen RL, Baccetti T. Changes in soft tissue nasal widths associated with rapid maxillary expansion in prepubertal and postpubertal subjects. *Angle Orthod.* 2010; 80(6): 995-1001.

[58] Iwasaki T, Saitoh I, Takemoto Y, Inada E, Kakuno E, Kanomi R, et al. Tongue posture improvement and pharyngeal airway enlargement as secondary effects of rapid maxillary expansion: a cone-beam computed tomography study. *Am J Orthod Dentofacial Orthop.* 2013; 143(2): 235-45.

[59] Ribeiro AN, de Paiva JB, Rinp-Neto J, Illipronti-Filho E, Trivino T, Fantini SM. Upper airway expansion after rapid maxillary expansion evaluated with cone beam computed tomography. *Angle Orthod.* 2012; 82(3): 458-63.

[60] Langer MRE, Itikawa CE, Valera FCP, Matsumoto MAN, Anselmo-Lima WT. Does rapid maxillary expansion increase nasopharyngeal space and improve nasal airway resistance? *Int J Pediatr Otorhinolaryngol.* 2011; 75: 122-5.

[61] Costa DJ, Mitchell R. Adenotonsillectomy for obstructive sleep apnea in obese children: a meta-analysis. *Otolaryngol Head Neck Surg* 2009; 140: 455-60.

http://dx.doi.org/10.5772/57885

[62] Marcus CL, Rosen G, Ward SL, Halbower AC, Sterni L, Lutz J, et al. Adherence to and effectiveness of positive airway pressure therapy in children with obstructive sleep apnea. Pediatrics. 2006; 117(3): e442-51.

Chapter 5

Swallowing, Gastroesophageal Reflux and Sleep Apnea

Shinji Teramoto

Additional information is available at the end of the chapter

http://dx.doi.org/10.5772/57577

1. Introduction

Because the pharynx is a shared conduit for swallowing and respiration, it is known that the breathing cycle is well coordinated with the swallowing in humans [1-3]. The process of inspiration and expiration is very precisely linked with the swallowing reflex via the supra-laryngeal nerve. However, the anatomical configuration of the pharynx may allow for the risk of food aspiration of material into the lower airways during bolus passage, particularly in elderly patients with a history of stroke and dementia [4-11]. The condition and function of the pharynx and upper airways may be considerably affected by nocturnal disturbed breathing including obstructive sleep apnea hypopnea syndrome (OSAHS) [12-14].

Gastro-esophageal reflux (GER) also affects the breathing and respiratory symptom [15]. The coincidence of recurrent respiratory symptoms and gastro-esophageal reflux (GER) is a well-known phenomenon in infants [16]. It has reported that gastro-esophageal reflux (GER) is increased in patients with OSAHS [15]. The GER is also associated with swallowing and breathing. Since the GER, OSAHS, and dysphagia are rapidly increased in adult and elderly patients, this chapter describes the interesting features of sleep apneas in terms of swallowing function and GER.

2. Breathing and swallowing

Swallowing function is necessary for eating, and it is coupled with breathing. it is well known that the breathing cycle is well coordinated with the swallowing in humans [1].The adult pattern of breathing-swallowing coordination during eating and drinking is well studied, with 75-95% of swallows beginning in the expiratory phase [2, 3] compared to 39% in newborns [4]. Swallowing elicits inspiratory suppression during breathing (Figure 1). Aspiration related infectious events are prevented by defense mechanisms, such as swallowing reflex, cough reflex, and mucocilliary clearance. Protection of the airway from aspiration requires inhibition of inspiratory airflow throughout the period of laryngeal exposure to the swallowed bolus. This respiratory inhibition is called deglutition apnea and appears to be a universal accompaniment of the normal swallow sequence in man [4-10]. Oral infusion of water at a variable rate of 40 ml/min while the subject breathes through the nose elicits repetitive swallows (rate: 8.1+/-4.1 swallows/min, mean+/-SD), but this does not cause a single incidence of coughing or aspiration in normal adults (Figure 2) [10]. The swallows interrupts inspiration and expiration and leads to compensatory changes in tidal volume and breathing frequency. Swallowing also causes respiratory phase resetting with a pattern that is characteristic of the strong perturbations of an attractor-cycle oscillator [11]. The threshold for initiation of swallowing in awake subjects is influenced by, but not strongly coupled to, the phase of respiration. The respiratory timing, in addition to anatomical barriers within the upper airway, influences the vulnerability for aspiration during deglutition. Swallows initiated near the expiratory-inspiratory transition may be the most likely to result in bolus aspiration, especially in pathological conditions that weaken the impact of swallowing on respiratory rhythm or slow the transport of the bolus through the pharynx [11]. Breathing and swallowing are well-controlled by the interaction of neuronal groups co-localized in the brainstem [12, 13]. This central neuronal control, combined with local anatomical conditions and sensory input from the pharynx, permit safe and directed passage of air and food materials. Ventilatory control as indicated by arterial partial pressure of CO2 affects swallowing [14, 15]. The dysphagia due to anatomical disorders or diseases may also affect breathing patterns [16-18]. The changes in pharyngeal function by surgical conditions may be concerned. However, the coupling between the swallowing and respiratory pattern generators is highly stable even in the post-laryngectomized patients [19].

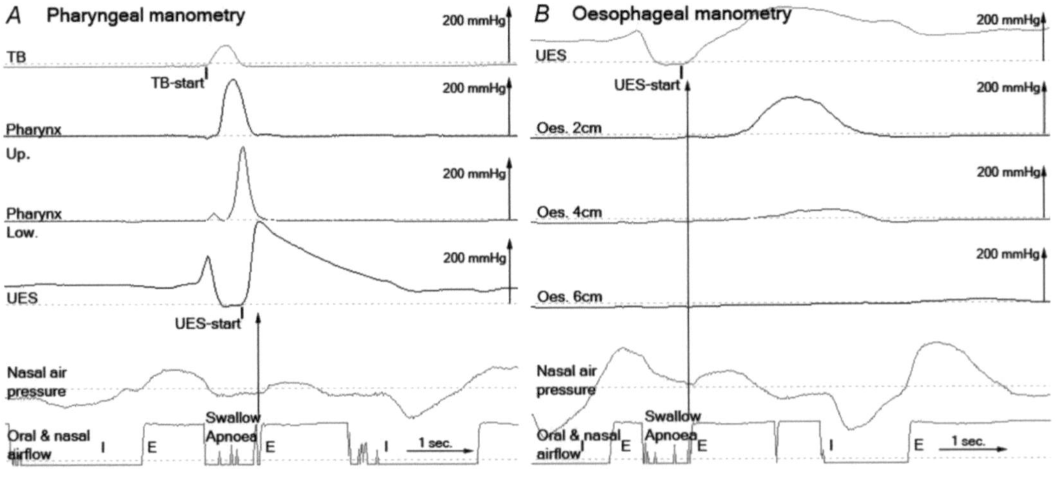

(cited by Hårdemark Cedborg A I et al. Exp Physiol 2009;94:459-468)

Figure 1. Pharyngeal and esophageal swallowing and swallowing apnea One swallow preceded and followed by expiration (respiratory phase pattern E–E). One swallow preceded and followed by expiration (respiratory phase pattern E–E). Recordings of pharyngeal (A) and oesophageal manometry (B), nasal air pressure and oral and nasal airflow by the bidirectional gas flow discriminator. The end of swallowing apnea is marked with arrows (↑). The start of pharyngeal swallowing is defined as the start of pressure rise at the tongue base (TB-start) and the end of pharyngeal swallowing as the start of pressure rise at the upper esophageal sphincter (UES-start), which also defines the start of the esophageal phase of swallowing. Pharyngeal manometry was recorded at the tongue base (TB), upper/lower level of the pharynx (Pharynx Up./Low.) and upper oesophageal sphincter (UES). Oesophageal manometry was recorded at 2, 4 and 6 cm below the UES. Inspiration (I), expiration (E).

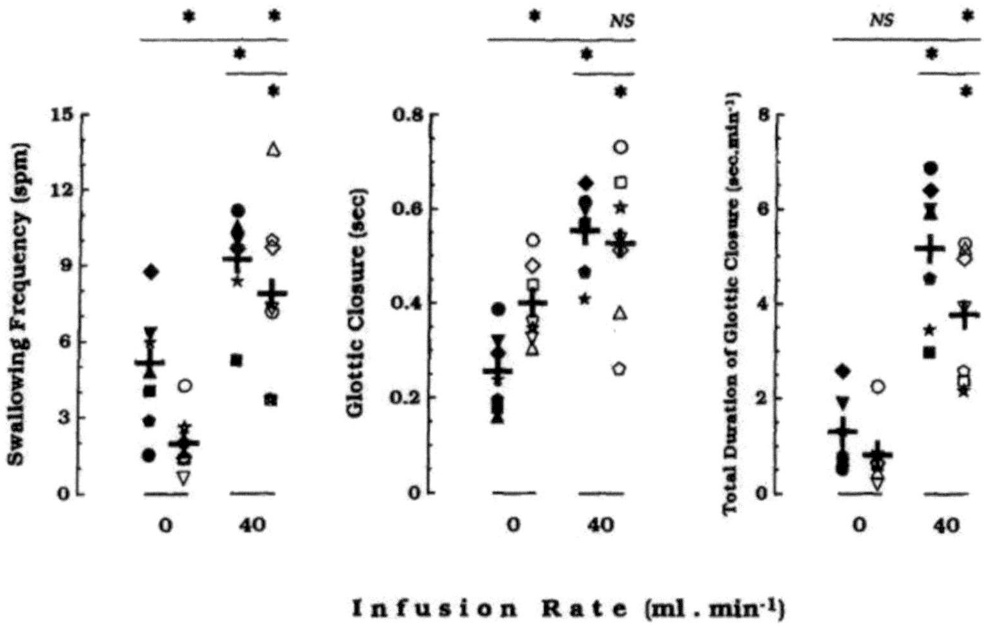

(Cited by Issa FG, Porostocky S. Control of ventilation during continuous swallowing. Am J Respir Crit Care Med 1994;150:1274-8.)

Figure 2. Changes in swallowing pattern during quiet breathing and CO_2 rebreathing. Swallowing pattern during quiet breathing (closed circles) and hypercapnic tests (open symbols) in control (no infusion, 0 mllmin) and continuous swallowing (40 ml/min) in seven subjects participating in the study. Different symbols represent mean data of different subjects, with bold crosses representing the mean data of all tests. Note that the number of swallows per minute (spm), duration of the swallow (glottic closure), and the total duration of glottic closure were higher during rebreathing tests than during control tests. Note also that the pattern of swallowing was different during quiet breathing than during CO2 rebreathing. Asterisks ($p < 0.05$) and NS (not significant) denote statistical difference between CO2 rebreathing and quiet breathing (top asterisks), between 40 and 0 infusion rates during quiet breathing (middle asterisks), and between 40 and 0 infusion ratesduring CO2 rebreathing (bottom asterisks).

3. Swallowing function in sleep apnea

The condition and function of the pharynx and upper airways is affected by nocturnal disturbed breathing and obstructive sleep apnea (OSA) [20]. Although the mechanisms of apnea termination in obstructive sleep apnea have not been fully elucidated, mechanoreceptor feedback from the respiratory muscles or pharynx has been thought to play an important role in apnea termination [21]. The influence of chemoreceptor information may be mediated indirectly through an effect on ventilatory effort. The constant positive airway pressure applied via a nose mask through the nares (nasal CPAP, nCPAP) has been established as the first line of therapy for obstructive sleep apnea hypopnea syndrome (OSAHS). It has been reported, however, that nCPAP exerts an inhibitory influence on the water-induced swallowing reflex [22].

Several investigators have reported that gastroesophageal reflux (GER) is increased in adult and child patients with OSAHS [23, 24]. It appears that the swallowing mechanism may be affected by mechanical and/or chemical stimuli, including apnea and positive pressures in the upper airways. Because abnormalities of neural networks in the area of the suprapharynx are implicated in the cause and/or results of obstructive sleep apneas, it is possible that patients with OSAHS have an abnormal swallowing reflex due to impaired neural/muscular function at the upper airways.

The phenomenon was observed. The swallowing reflex was determined according to the following criteria: latent time (LT), the time following a bolus injection of distilled water at the suprapharynx to the onset of swallowing; inspiratory suppression time (IST), the time from the termination of swallowing to the next onset of inspiration; and threshold volume, the minimum volume of water (range, 0.4 to 2 mL) that could evoke the swallowing response. Whereas the LT values in patients with OSAS were larger than the LT values in the control subjects, the IST values (which may reflect the switching mechanism from deglutition apnea to breathing) were actually shorter (Figure 3). In addition, a greater bolus volume was necessary to elicit swallowing in patients with OSAHS than was necessary in the control subjects. Thus, patients with OSAHS are likely to exhibit an impaired swallowing reflex, probably due to the perturbed neural and muscular function of the upper airways [25]. However, Jobin and others have reported that threshold volume did not differ between the OSAHS and control groups with obesity. Although the swallowing latency was shorter for OSA patients, IST were similar for OSA patients and control subjects. Since there was a significant inverse relation between vibratory sensation threshold (VST) and IST, oropharyngeal sensory impairment in OSA may be associated with an attenuation of inhibitory modulating inputs to reflex and central control of upper airway swallowing function [26].

4. Clinical implication of swallowing dysfunction in sleep apnea

Sleep apnea caused swallowing dysfunction may lead to susceptibility to upper airway infection in child patients and older patients [27-29]. The increased respiratory effort to breath against a closed airway may facilitate pulmonary aspiration in the patients. It is known that children with sleep-disordered breathing experience more respiratory infections. Sleep apnea associated swallowing abnormality is possibly a predisposing risk factor for community-acquired pneumonia (CAP) in children [27]. In the frail elderly, sleep apnea considered to be a significant risk factor for the development of pneumonia [28-30]. Further, immune perturbations secondary to disrupted sleep may render them susceptible to invasion of pathogens [31]. The impaired immune function caused by sleep-disturbed breathing may also potentiate the emergence of pneumonia.

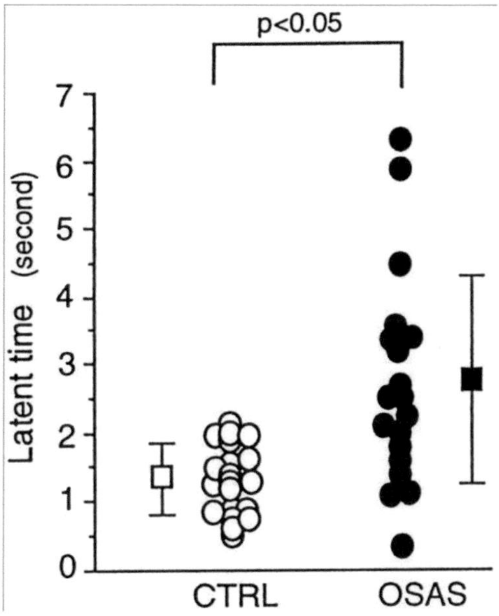

(Cited by Teramoto et al. Chest Chest. 1999;116(1):17-21. doi:10.1378/chest.116.1.17)

Figure 3. Swallowing reflex in OSAS patients and control subjects. A presentation of the latency for the swallowing reflex induced by a bolus of water in 20 patients with OSAS and in 20 age-matched control subjects (CTRL). The latency for swallowing initiation was judged using LT on the recording of submental EMG activity.

From treatment viewpoints of sleep apnea, nCPAP therapy may have favorable effects on the risk reduction of airway infection. The treatment of OSAHS with CPAP may be effective for the improvement of awakens and daytime activity as well as the prevention of nocturnal aspiration and pneumonia. On the other hand, poor maintenance of the CPAP machine and the humidifier leads to bacterial growth. Although this does not cause an infection, it can result in the introduction of bacteria to the patient's respiratory system. Keeping the machine and its components clean decreases the opportunity for bacterial growth. The only infection clearly associated with CPAP use may be meningitis. It has been reported that meningitis occurred in patients using CPAP only following a skull trauma [31]. In the elderly, OSA and central type apnea was associated with an increase in mortality from pneumonia in addition to increased risk of cardiovascular related and all-cause mortality. However, there was no relationship between mortality and severity of sleep apnea [32].

5. Breathing and gastroesophageal reflux (GER)

Acid reflux events are very different between the awake period and the sleep period. During sleep, acid reflux events tend to be less frequent and of a longer duration as compared with acid reflux events during the awake period [33]. This is due to the profound effect of sleep on esophageal response to acid reflux events. During sleep, there is a significant reduction in voluntary swallowing and thus primary peristalsis. In addition, diminished saliva production during sleep results in delayed normalization of the distal esophageal pH after an acid reflux event has occurred. Loss of gravitation effect as well as alteration in perception of acid reflux events and thus less symptom generation may all adversely affect physiological response to GER. Consequently, nocturnal GER has been demonstrated to be associated with esophageal inflammation, GER-related complications and extra-esophageal manifestations of gastroesophageal reflux disease (GERD) [34, 35]. It is well known that GERD, besides its classical symptoms, is associated with extra esophageal symptoms and complications as well (Table 1). The most common ones are respiratory symptoms, no cardiac chest pain, and physiatrist symptoms including nocturnal disturbed breathing [36-38].

Organ specialty	Symptoms /complications
Cardiology	non-cardiac chest pain
Pulmonologist	bronchial asthma, chronic cough
Otolaryngology	Posterior laryngitis, reflux laryngitis,
Psychiatry	sleep disorders, sexual disorders, anxiety
Pediatrics	recurrent lower respiratory tract infection, apnea (sudden death), otitis media
Geriatrics	sleep disorders, recurrent lower respiratory tract infection

Table 1. Extra-esophageal complications of GERD

6. Gastroesophageal reflux in sleep apnea

Gastroesophageal reflux disease (GERD) is a very common disorder defined as various symptoms or esophageal mucosal damage generated by the abnormal reflux of gastric contents into the esophagus [39]. Patients with OSAHS have been reported to have a high prevalence of gastroesophageal reflux (GER) symptoms [40]. The increase of transdiaphragmatic pressure in parallel with the large negative intrathoracic pressure produced during apnea events may directly lead to GER (Figure 4) [41]. Some studies have demonstrated that the application of nCPAP for OSAHS also improve GER symptoms. However, GER does not occur with every apnea [42]. Because the common conditions observed in patients with OSAHS, including obesity or alcohol ingestion, are also predisposing factors for GER, the direct pathologic association between OSAHS and GER has not been established. In fact, a recent investigation in over 1000 subjects failed to show a causal link between both diseases [43]. Thus, there is a common pathology between OSAHS and GERD, but the direct causal relationships between two disorders remains controversial. Further, a temporal relationship between cough and reflux events has been suggested by studies utilizing impedance-pH monitoring of reflux events and objective cough recording. However, consensus is lacking in terms of whether this temporal relationship proves a causal link between reflux and cough [44].

http://dx.doi.org/10.5772/57577

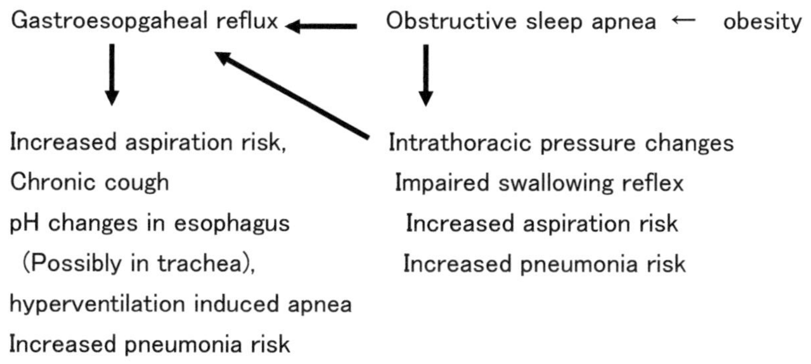

Figure 4. Possible pathologic link between gastroesopgaheal reflux (GER) and sleep apnea

7. Clinical implication of GER in sleep apnea

Extraesophageal complications of GERD have been concerned in patients with sleep apnea. The GER may be associated with cardiovascular, pulmonologic, laryngeal, and dental complications [45]. The most recognized manifestations are non-cardiac chest pain, bronchial asthma, chronic bronchitis, chronic cough, and posterior laryngitis, as well as the acidic damage of dental enamel [45].

Heartburn during sleep is very common in the general population. This type of symptom of GERD is strongly associated with increased body mass index (BMI), carbonated soft drink consumption, snoring, daytime sleepiness, insomnia, hypertension, bronchial asthma, and usage of benzodiazepines. These factors are also strong risk factors for sleep apnea. Thus, heartburn during sleep may be associated with the severity of OSA related negative intra-thoracic pressure, resulting in increased sleep complaints and excessive daytime sleepiness [46]. It has been suggested that sleep deprivation is hyperalgesic in patients with GERD and provides a potential mechanism for increase in GERD symptom severity in sleep-deprived patients [47].

8. Possible links among dysphagia, GER and sleep apnea

Chronic cough is a common problem in patients who visit physicians. The cough is associated with deterioration in patients' quality of life. The three most common causes of chronic cough in those who are referred to pulmonary specialists are postnasal drip, asthma and gastroeso-phageal reflux. It has been reported that asthma, postnasal drip syndrome (PNDS), and gastroesophageal reflux disease (GERD), alone or in combination, were responsible for > 90% of the causes of chronic cough [48]. The chronic cough may lead to true asthma and asthma is exacerbated by the gastroesopgaeal reflux [49, 50]. The initial treatment of patients with cough is often empiric and may involve a trial of decongestants, bronchodilators or histamine H2 antagonists, as monotherapy or in combination [51]. If a therapeutic trial is not successful, sequential diagnostic testing including chest radiograph, and barium swallow may be indicated. The chronic cough could be caused by repeated GER, aspiration, and OSA [52]. The pathologic link between chronic cough and sleep apneas has been considered. The chronic cough is a symptom of GER and dysphagia. The daytime symptom may affect the night time symptom including sleep apneas. One possible explanation for the risk of chronic cough in OSA patients may be related to easy pulmonary aspiration. Since high collapsibility of the upper airway is characteristic to OSA, resultant hypoxemia may stimulate such patients to breath against a closed airway, therefore generating a more negative intra-thoracic pressure [53-55]. The more negative intra-thoracic pressure induces a higher pressure gradient and a vacuum pressure through the upper airway, facilitating aspiration of pharyngeal secretions, saliva or oral contents into the lower respiratory tract[56]. Because the fundamental mechanism of sleep-disordered breathing in children may not be the same as that of sleep apneas in adults and the elderly, the inter-relationships among chronic cough, sleep apnea, and GER in younger subjects and children is different from those in adult and elderly patients. Post-swallow apnea and post-swallow inspiration occur significantly more frequently in infants suffering from acute bronchiolitis than healthy infants [57].It is interesting to know the swallowing function in child patients and older patients with sleep apneas or GERD. Because the swallowing function is impaired in patients with OSAHS, and because the swallowing function is associated with cough reflex thorough substance P, the abnormality in swallowing function in OSAS may be associated with chronic cough in children and adults [58, 59]. It has been suggested that excessive daytime sleepiness seen in some OSAHS patients may be associated with various pathophysiological mechanisms including changes in substance P levels [60]. Although many patients with adults OSAHS complain of sleep-related heartburn and regurgitation of gastric contents into the pharynx, the complaint is rarely heard in children with apneas. Therefore, the similarities and differences in swallowing function, cough reflex, and GER between children and adult patients with SAS may lead to further knowledge regarding the coupling mechanism between respiration and deglutition [61, 53]. However, as GERD manifests a spectrum of conditions, including asthma, posterior laryngitis, and chronic coughing, the pathologic link among chronic cough, OSAS, and GERD is not simply determined in children.

9. Summary

Breathing and swallowing is tightly coupled. Disruption of breathing-swallowing coordination causes aspiration, which facilitates several pulmonary complications including lower respiratory tract infection.

Swallowing is also affected by the gastroesophageal reflux (GER). Thus, GER affects respiratory symptom including aspiration, cough, and dysphasia. The coincidence of recurrent respiratory symptoms and GER is important in infants as well as elderly patients. The GER related respiratory symptoms are considerably influenced by nocturnal disturbed breathing including OSAHS. The intrathoracic pressure changes during obstructive apnea and compensated hyperinflation are associated with the occurrence of GER and aspiration. We should seriously consider that the swallowing, breathing and GER are dependently and independently linked in various clinical condition during daytime and nighttime.

Author details

Shinji Teramoto*

Address all correspondence to: shinjit-tky@umin.ac.jp

Department of Pulmonary Medicine, Hitachinaka Medical Education and Research Center, Graduate School of Comprehensive Human Sciences, University of Tsukuba, Japan

References

[1] Smith J, Wolkove N, Colacone A, et al. Coordination of eating, drinking and breathing in adults. Chest 1989; 96:578–582

[2] Preiksaitis HG, Mayrand S, Robins K, Diamant NE. Coordination of respiration and swallowing: effect of bolus volume in normal adults. Am J Physiol 1992; 263(3 Pt 2), R624-630.

[3] Hiss SG, Treole K, Stuart A.Effects of age, gender, bolus volume, and trial on swallowing apnea duration and swallow/respiratory phase relationships of normal adults. Dysphagia, 2001; 16(2): 128-135.

[4] Bamford O, Taciak V, Gewolb IH. The relationship between rhythmic swallowing and breathing during suckle feeding in term neonates. Pediatr Res, 1992;31(6): 619-624.

[5] Wilson SL, Thach BT, Brouillette RT, Abu-Osba YK. Coordination of breathing and swallowing in human infants. Journal of Applied Physiology, 1981;50: 851-858.

[6] Nishino T, Yonezawa T, Honda Y. Effects of swallowing on the pattern of continuous respiration in human adults. Am Rev Respir Dis. 1985;132(6):1219-22.

[7] Selley WG, Flack FC, Ellis RE, Brooks WA. Respiratory patterns associated with swallowing: Part 1. The normal adult pattern and changes with age. Age Ageing. 1989;18(3):168-72.

[8] Nishino T, Tanaka A, Ishikawa T, Hiraga K. Respiratory, laryngeal, and tracheal responses to nasal insufflation of volatile anesthetics in anesthetized humans. Anesthesiology. 1991;75:441-444.

[9] Shaker R, Li Q, Ren J, Townsend WF, Dodds WJ, Martin BJ, et al. Coordination of deglutition and phases of respiration: effect of aging, tachypnea, bolus volume, and chronic obstructive pulmonary disease. Am J Physiol, 1992;263: G750-755.

[10] Issa FG, Porostocky S. Control of ventilation during continuous swallowing. Am J Respir Crit Care Med. 1994;150:1274-1278.

[11] Paydarfar D, Gilbert RJ, Poppel CS, et al. Respiratory phase resetting and airflow changes induced by swallowing in humans. J Physiol (Lond) 1995; 483:273–288

[12] Dick TE, Oku Y, Romaniuk JR & Cherniack NS.Interaction between central pattern generators for breathing and swallowing in the cat. J Physiol 1993; 465, 715–730.

[13] Saito Y, Ezure K, Tanaka I. Swallowing-related activities of respiratory and non-respiratory neurons in the nucleus of solitary tract in the rat. J Physiol 2002; 540: 1047–1060.

[14] Sai T, Isono S, Nishino T. Effects of withdrawal of phasic lung inflation during normocapnia and hypercapnia on the swallowing reflex in humans. J Anesth 2004; 18: 82–88.

[15] Nishino T, Hasegawa R, Ide T, Isono S. Hypercapnia enhances the development of coughing during continuous infusion of water into the pharynx. Am J Respir Crit Care Med 1998; 157, 815–821.

[16] Nilsson H, Ekberg O, Bülow M, Hindfelt B. Assessment of respiration during video fluoroscopy of dysphagic patients. Acad Radiol 1997; 4: 503–507.

[17] Hadjikoutis S, Pickersgill TP, Dawson K, Wiles CM. Abnormal patterns of breathing during swallowing in neurological disorders. Brain 2000;123, 1863–1873.

[18] Terzi N, Orlikowski D, Aegerter P, Lejaille M, Ruquet M, Zalcman G, Fermanian C, Raphael JC, Lofaso F. Breathing–swallowing interaction in neuromuscular patients: a physiological evaluation. Am J Respir Crit Care Med 2007; 175: 269–276.

[19] Charbonneau I, Lund JP, McFarland DH.-Persistence of respiratory-swallowing coordination after laryngectomy. Journal of Speech, Language and Research 2005; 48: 34-44

[20] Radwan L, Maszczyk Z, Koziorowski A, Koziej M, Cieslicki J, Sliwinski P, Zielinski J. Control of breathing in obstructive sleep apnea and in patients with the overlap syndrome. Eur Respir J 1995; 8:542–545

[21] Kimoff RJ, Cheong TH, Olha AE, Charbonneau M, Levy RD, Cosio MG, Gottfried SB. Mechanisms of apnea termination in obstructive sleep apnea. Role of chemoreceptor and mechanoreceptor stimuli. Am J Respir Crit Care Med. 1994;149:707-714.

[22] Nishino T, Sugimori K, Kohchi A, Hiraga K. Nasal constant positive airway pressure inhibits the swallowing reflex. Am Rev Respir Dis. 1989;140:1290-3.

[23] Ing AJ, Ngu MC, Breslin AB. Obstructive sleep apnea and gastroesophageal reflux. Am J Med. 2000;108 Suppl 4a:120S-125S.

[24] Noronha AC, de Bruin VM, Nobre e Souza MA, de Freitas MR, Araújo Rde P, Mota RM, de Bruin PF. Gastroesophageal reflux and obstructive sleep apnea in childhood. Int J Pediatr Otorhinolaryngol. 2009;73:383-389.

[25] Teramoto S, Sudo E, Matsuse T, Ohga E, Ishii T, Ouchi Y, Fukuchi Y. Impaired swallowing reflex in patients with obstructive sleep apnea syndrome. Chest. 1999;116:17-21.

[26] Jobin V, et al, Swallowing function and upper airway sensation in obstructive sleep apnea. J Appl Physiol 2007; 102:1587–1594

[27] Goldbart AD, Tal A, Givon-Lavi N, Bar-Ziv J, Dagan R, Greenberg D. Sleep-disordered breathing is a risk factor for community-acquired alveolar pneumonia in early childhood. Chest. 2012;141:1210-1215.

[28] Ishii M, Yamaguchi Y, Yamamoto H, Ouchi Y, Osumi S, Nakamura T. Relationship between sleep apnea and respiratory infections in bedridden elderly individuals on tube feeding. J Am Geriatr Soc. 2012 ;60:790-792

[29] Sanner BM, Fluerenbrock N, Kleiber-Imbeck A, et al. Effect of continuous positive airway pressure therapy on infectious complications in patients with obstructive sleep apnea syndrome. Respiration 2001;68:483-487

[30] Morimoto S, Takahashi T, Okaishi K, Okuro M, Nakahashi T, Sakamoto D, Mizuno T, Kanda T, Takahashi M, Toga H. Sleep apnoea syndrome as a risk for mortality in elderly inpatients. J Int Med Res 2012;40:601-11.

[31] Besedovsky L, Lange T, Born J. Sleep and immune function. Pflugers Arch 2012;463:121-137

[32] Kuzniar TJ, Gruber B, Mutlu GM. Cerebrospinal fluid leak and meningitis associated with nasal continuous positive airway pressure therapy. Chest. 2005;128:1882-1884.

[33] Orr W, Johnson L, Robinson M. Effect of sleep on swallowing, esophageal peristalsis, and acid clearance. Gastroenterology 1984; 86: 814–819.

[34] Cuttitta G, Cibella F, Visconti A, et al. Spontaneous gastroesophageal reflux and airway patency during the night in adult asthmatics. Am J Respir Crit Care Med 2000; 161: 177–181

[35] Jacob P, Kahrilas P, Herzon G. Proximal esophageal pH-metry in patients with 'reflux laryngitis'. Gastroenterology 1991; 100: 305–310.

[36] Demeter P, Pap A. The relationship between gastroesophageal reflux disease and obstructive sleep apnea.-J Gastroenterol 2004;39:815-820

[37] Teramoto S, Ohga E, Matsui H, et al. Obstructive sleep apnea syndrome may be a significant cause of gastroesophageal reflux disease in older people.J Am Geriatr Soc1999;47, 1273-1274

[38] Teramoto S, Yamamoto H, Ouchi Y. Gastroesophageal reflux is common in patients with sleep apnea rather than snorers without sleep apnea. Chest 2003;124:767-768.

[39] ltomare A, Guarino MP, Cocca S, Emerenziani S, Cicala M. Gastroesophageal reflux disease: Update on inflammation and symptom perception. World J Gastroenterol. 2013;19(39):6523-6528.

[40] Guilleminault C. Obstructive sleep apnea: the clinical syndrome and historical perspective. Med Clin North Am 1985;69:1187–1203,

[41] Kerr P, Shoenut JP, Millar T, Buckle P, Kryger MH. Nasal CPAP reduces gastroesophageal reflux in obstructive sleep apnea syndrome. Chest. 1992;101:1539-1544.

[42] Penzel T, Becker H, Brandenburg U, et al. Arousal in patients with gastro-oesophageal reflux and sleep apnoea. Eur Respir J 1999; 14:1266–1270

[43] MizutaY, Takeshima F, Shikuwa S, Ikeda S, Kohno S. Is there a specific linkage between obstructive sleep apnea syndrome and gastroesophageal reflux disease ? Digestive Endoscopy 2006;18: 88–97

[44] Kahrilas PJ, Smith JA, Dicpinigaitis PV. A Causal Relationship Between Cough and Gastroesophageal Reflux Disease (GERD) has been Established: A Pro/Con Debate. Lung. 2013 Nov 13. (Epub ahead of print)

[45] Poelmans J, Tack J. Extraoesophageal manifestations of gastro-oesophageal reflux. Gut. 2005;54:1492–9.

[46] Bytzer P. Assessment of reflux symptom severity: methodological options and their attributes. Gut. 2004;53:iv28–34.

[47] Fass R, Quan SF, O'Connor GT, Ervin A, Iber C. Predictors of heartburn during sleep in a large prospective cohort study. Chest 2005;127:1658-66.

[48] Schey R, Dickman R, Parthasarathy S, Quan SF, Wendel C, Merchant J, Powers J, Han B, van Handel D, Fass R. Sleep deprivation is hyperalgesic in patients with gastroesophageal reflux disease. Gastroenterology. 2007;133:1787-95.

[49] Palombini, BC, Villanova, CAC, Araujo, E, et al. A pathologic triad in chronic cough: asthma, postnasal drip syndrome, and gastroesophageal reflux disease.Chest 1999; 116: 279-284.

[50] Stein, MR Advances in the approach to gastroesophageal reflux (GER) and asthma.J Asthma1999;36, 309-314.

[51] Bruno, G, Graf, U, Andreozzi, P Gastric asthma: an unrecognized disease with an unsuspected frequency.J Asthma1999;36, 315-325.

[52] Irwin RS, Madison JM: The Diagnosis and Treatment of Cough, N. Eng. J. Med, 343, 1715-1721, 2000

[53] Teramoto S, Ouchi Y. A possible pathologic link between chronic cough and sleep apnea syndrome through gastroesophageal reflux disease in older people. Chest 2000; 117(4):1215-1216.

[54] Morrell MJ, Arabi Y, Zahn B, et al. Progressive retropalatal narrowing preceding obstructive apnea. Am J Respir Crit Care Med 1998;158:1974-1981

[55] Schwab RJ, Gupta KB, Gefter WB, et al. Upper airway and soft tissue anatomy in normal subjects and patients with sleep-disordered breathing:Significance of the lateral pharyngeal walls. Am J Respir Crit Care Med 1995;152:1673-1689

[56] Schwab RJ, Pasirstein M, Pierson R, et al. Identification of upper airway anatomic risk factors for obstructive sleep apnea with volumetric magnetic resonance imaging. Am J Respir Crit Care Med 2003;168:522-530

[57] Dempsey JA, Veasey SC, Morgan BJ, et al. Pathophysiology of sleep apnea. Physiol Rev 2010;90:47-112

[58] Pinnington L L, Smith CM, Ellis RE, Morton RE. Feeding efficiency and respiratory integration respiratory integration in infants with acute viral bronchiolitis. J Pediatrics, 2000;137:523-526.

[59] Sekizawa, K, Ujiie, Y, Itabashi, S, et al Lack of cough reflex in patients with aspiration pneumonia(letter).Lancet1990;335, 1228-1229

[60] Hatipoğlu U. Rubinstein I. Inflammation and Obstructive Sleep Apnea Syndrome Pathogenesis: A Working Hypothesis. Respiration 2003;70:665–671

[61] Ursavas A. Upregulating substance P levels to treat obstructive sleep apnea. Expert Opin Ther Targets. 2008;12:583-8.

Chapter 6

COPD and Sleep Apnea Syndrome – Impact and Interaction of Coexisting Disease

Carlos Zamarrón Sanz, Carlos Rábade Castedo,
Ester Zamarrón de Lucas, Emilio Morete Aracay and
Félix del Campo Matias

Additional information is available at the end of the chapter

http://dx.doi.org/10.5772/57594

1. Introduction

Chronic obstructive pulmonary disease (COPD), a common preventable and treatable disease, is characterized by persistent airflow limitation that is usually progressive and associated with an enhanced chronic inflammatory response in the airways and the lung to noxious particles or gases (Global Strategy for the Diagnosis, 2013).

The chronic airflow limitation characteristic of COPD is caused by a mixture of small-airway disease (obstructive bronchiolitis) and parenchymal destruction (emphysema). The relative contributions of each vary from person to person. Chronic inflammation causes structural changes and narrowing of the small airways.

Symptoms of COPD include sputum production, cough and dyspnea. These respiratory symptoms are chronic and progressive over time. As a result, subjects increasingly experience deterioration in their health-related quality of life, in their capacity to work and reduced participation in social and physical activities (Rabe et al., 2007).

COPD includes heterogeneous lesions that variably affect the airways, lung parenchyma and systemic structures. COPD is caused by various pathogenic mechanisms and does not present a uniform histological substrate. Patients with this disease present with different clinical features: non-exacerbator with emphysema or chronic bronchitis; mixed COPD-asthma; exacerbator with emphysema and exacerbator with chronic bronchitis (Miravitlles et al., 2013). In addition to affecting the lungs, the disease presents significant systemic consequences including skeletal muscle dysfunction, nutritional disorders and weight loss (Andreassen &

Vestbo, 2003; Agusti, 2005). As a result COPD causes a progressive decrease in the ability to perform the essential activities of daily living.

COPD is a leading cause of morbidity and mortality worldwide and results in an economic and social burden that is both considerable and increasing. According to some studies, the prevalence of COPD in Spain is 10.6% (Sobradillo et al., 1999), and the mortality rate in 2011 was 51.2 deaths per 100,000 males and 14.6 deaths per 100,000 females (Instituto Nacional de Estadística, 2011).

Due to its high prevalence, morbidity and mortality, COPD generates significant economic costs to the health system and is considered a significant health problem.

Obstructive sleep apnea syndrome (OSAS) is a disorder characterized by recurrent upper airway collapse during sleep (Young et al., 1993). This results in a reduction or complete cessation of airflow despite ongoing inspiratory efforts and leads to arousals, sleep fragmentation, and oxyhemoglobin desaturation (Remmers et al., 1978).

OSAS is a common disease, affecting 3.4% in men and 3% in women of the adult population and appears to be associated with a number of forms of morbidity (Duran et al., 2001). Al least 6.8% of subjects 50-70 years of age are affected (Zamarron et al., 1999).

The most common symptoms of OSAS patients include chronic loud snoring, excessive daytime sleepiness, personality changes and deterioration of quality of life. Though clinically recognized for more than three decades (Gastaut et al., 1965; Lugaresi et al., 1972; Guilleminault, 1985), general awareness of OSAS has been slow to develop.

Treatment with continuous positive airway pressure (CPAP) has been shown to decrease the frequency and severity of sleep disturbances and associated symptoms (Kiely et al., 1999). Other treatments include mandibular advancement prosthesis (Doff et al., 2013) or surgery (Tuncel et al., 2012).

OSAS may coexist with COPD and this combination has been the focus of extensive study. Fenley referred to it as ''overlap syndrome'' (Flenley, 1985). Recently, to encourage further research in this area, another terminology has been proposed to integrate OSAS in the setting of obstructive lung disease, which is called OLDOSA (obstructive lung disease and obstructive sleep apnea) (Ioachimescu & Teodorescu, 2013).

The aim of the present review is to analyse the association and interaction of obstructive sleep apnea syndrome and chronic obstructive lung disease.

2. Epidemiology

There have been a number of studies evaluating the presence of OSAS among COPD patients. Chaouat et al. found a 14% prevalence of OSAS among patients with mild COPD (Chaouat et al., 1995), and O'Brien found overlap syndrome in 11.9% of COPD patients (O'Brien & Whitman, 2005).

On the other hand, there have also been studies evaluating the presence of COPD among patients with OSAS. In a group of 265 OSAS patients, Chaouat found that 11% also had COPD (Chaouat et al., 1995). Sanders et al. found 11% of overlap syndrome among patients with OSAS (Sanders et al., 2003). Nevertheless, a very large study including 5,954 participants done in conjunction with the Sleep Heart Health Study found no significant difference in the prevalence of OSAS, defined as apnea hypopnea index greater than 10, among COPD subjects (14.0%) and those without COPD (18.6%) (Sanders et al., 2003). A study involving 356 males and 320 females with OSAS found a lower prevalence of overlap syndrome (9.2%) (Bednarek et al., 2005). Recently, in 524 male subjects with OSAS diagnosed by the prevalence rate of COPD was 12% (Shiina et al., 2012).

All of this suggests that the coexistence of COPD and OSAS is due more to chance than a pathophysiologic link between the two conditions.

Among the different phenotypes that constitute COPD, OSAS is preferably associated to chronic bronchitis. Study results COPDGene showed that patients with chronic bronchitis phenotype showed prevalence of OSAS 22.4% versus 14.4% in those who did not meet this criterion (Kim et al., 2011). These findings are consistent with the idea that the chronic bronchitis patient may present episodic nocturnal desaturations during REM sleep. Izquierdo et al. also found that the prevalence of OSAS is more prevalent in the phenotype chronic bronchitis and emphysema, compared to COPD and asthma (23.6, 4.9% and 12.5%, respectively (Izquierdo-Alonso et al., 2013).

3. Physiopatological consequences

Sleep has profound effects on ventilation (Douglas et al., 1982), partly because it is accompanied by a fall in metabolic rate (White et al., 1985). Sleep represents a challenge to the respiratory system, especially in patients debilitated by respiratory disease. As occurs in some respiratory diseases, patients affected by respiratory failure while awake, are even more seriously affected during sleep.

In overlap syndrome, ventilatory response may be disturbed by lung mechanics and gas exchange. Radwan et al. studied breathing pattern and CO_2 response in obese patients with overlap syndrome and obese patients with OSAS only. The OSAS group presented similar values to non-obese controls in ventilatory response to CO_2 and occlusion pressure responses. The overlap group had a higher breathing frequency and lower tidal volume than the OSAS-only group. This author concluded that overlap patients with hypercapnia had both blunted ventilatory and mouth occlusion pressure responses during CO_2. In patients with chronic hypercapnia, there is an increased blood bicarbonate concentration, which may inhibit CO_2 sensitivity and decreases mouth occlusion pressure response (Radwan et al., 1995).

In patients with overlap syndrome, sleep-related hypoventilation is associated to a reduction in respiratory drive, loss of accessory muscle activity and ventilation perfusion mismatch. Hypoventilation in such patients is due to an increased breathing effort, related to upper and lower airway obstruction. Respiratory muscles may also fatigue which is related to the mechanical disadvantage of chest wall hyperinflation. Moreover, there is also a reduction in functional residual capacity which is related to supine posture and sleep state (McNicholas, 1997). Kwon et al. suggest that increased severity of hyperinflation is associated with worse sleep efficiency, independent of apnea and nocturnal hypoxemia. The mechanisms underlying this observation are uncertain. These authors speculate that therapies aimed at reducing lung hyperinflation may improve sleep quality in patients with overlap syndrome (Kwon et al., 2009).

Overlap patients present more nocturnal desaturation than patients with either OSAS or COPD alone (Chaouat et al., 1995; Sanders et al., 2003). Sanders examined the degree to which COPD and OSAS independently and jointly contribute to desaturation during sleep. After adjusting for age, sex, height, weight, race, smoking status, and awake oxygen saturation, the OR for nocturnal oxyhemoglobin desaturation was found to be considerably increased in OSAS patients (Sanders et al., 2003). Furthermore, Lacedonia suggest that day-time hypoxemia in overlap patients is largely determined by the increase of body weight and severity of nocturnal hypoxia (Lacedonia et al., 2013).

4. Pulmonary hypertension

Patients with overlap syndrome are more likely to develop daytime pulmonary hypertension (Weitzenblum et al., 1988) and right heart failure (Bradley & Phillipson, 1985) than patients with either condition alone. COPD patients are affected by pulmonary hypertension secondary to alveolar hypoxia (Bonsignore et al., 1994), which is associated to increased morbidity and mortality (Chaouat et al., 2005). In these patients, pulmonary hypertension is primarily observed in those with severe disease, when the FEV_1 is lower than 50% predicted and diurnal PaO_2 is less than 60 mm Hg (Ashutosh et al., 1983).

OSAS patients may also be affected by pulmonary hypertension (Bady et al., 2000). However, this impact is higher when associated with COPD. In fact, Hawrylkiewicz et al. found a prevalence of pulmonary hypertension among overlap patients of 80% compared to 16% among individuals with OSAS alone (Hawrylkiewicz et al., 2004).

Patients with simultaneous COPD and OSAS have a more serious sleep related oxygen desaturacion than patients with COPD alone and the same degree of bronchial obstruction. Chaouat et al. reported a $PaO2 \leq 65$ mm Hg in 54 (23%) out of 235 non-OSAS COPD patients and compared to 17 (57%) out of 30 patients with overlap syndrome (Chaouat et al., 1995). In the same report, right-heart catheterization identified pulmonary hypertension in 7% of patients with COPD and 36% of those with overlap syndrome. In fact, hypoxemia, hypercapnia, and pulmonary hypertension were observed in the presence of even mild to moderate bronchial obstruction in overlap patients (Fletcher et al., 1987). When COPD reaches an advanced-stage, concomitant OSAS is likely to cause significant adverse clinical consequences (Hiestand & Phillips, 2008).

5. Sleep apnea syndrome and COPD association and vascular disease

COPD is a systemic disease with multiple effects on target-organs including cardiovascular system. Until recently, exacerbations of disease and progression of respiratory insufficiency have been the focus of mortality studies in COPD, however, a number of epidemiologic reports have shown that significant morbidity and mortality in COPD involves cardiovascular diseases.

In France, Fuhrman et al found that cardiovascular disease accounted for 32% of deaths in COPD patients (Fuhrman et al., 2006). Similar results were obtained in previous retrospective studies conducted in Canada (Huiart et al., 2005; Curkendall et al., 2006). In these reports, cardiovascular morbidity and mortality were higher in the COPD group than in the general population.

Moreover, some prospective reports have shown that FEV_1 is a factor that predicts mortality risk from all causes and specifically mortality from ischemic heart disease in both genders independently of the smoking habit (Schunemann et al., 2000). In Spain, De Lucas-Ramos et al. in a cross sectional multicentre study of 572 COPD patients found a prevalence of 16.4% of ischemic heart disease (De Lucas-Ramos et al., 2008). In a subsequent paper of 1200 COPD patients and 300 control subjects, these authors found that COPD was an independent risk factor for cardiovascular disease with an odds ratio of 2.23 (1.18 to 4.24) (De Lucas-Ramos et al., 2012). However, Izquierdo et al, in another case-control study found no association between ischemic heart disease and COPD and concluded that the higher prevalence of traditional cardiovascular risk factors in patients with COPD may explain the higher incidence of ischemic heart disease in these patients (Izquierdo et al., 2010).

A close relationship exists between COPD, systemic inflammation and cardiovascular disease, but the mechanisms by which COPD patients develop systemic inflammation remain unclear. Although the main abnormality favouring vascular disease associated with COPD is systemic inflammation, other factors include the activation of platelets related to hypoxia and oxidative stress (Takabatake et al., 2000; Mills et al., 2008). In COPD there is a systemic inflammatory component which manifests itself in the presence of several inflammatory mediators in peripheral blood (Gan et al., 2004).

An extensively-studied inflammatory mediator is C-reactive protein. Studies have shown that patients with COPD have higher values of C-reactive protein and that these are independent of smoking (Pinto-Plata et al., 2006; Karadag et al., 2008). C-reactive protein exerts diverse effects on endothelial biology by promoting proinflammatory and proatherogenic phenotype, currently considered to be a systemic marker of the inflammatory process associated with cardiovascular disease.

It has also been found that homocysteine in blood, another marker for cardiovascular disease, was elevated in severe stable COPD patients (Seemungal et al., 2007). In a three-year follow-up study of a cohort of 3247 subjects, Nunomiya et al. found that levels of homocysteine in blood were predictive of FEV_1 reduction (Nunomiya et al., 2013). In addition, elevated levels of inflammatory markers such as TNF-alpha, IL-6, IL-8 have also been reported in patients with COPD (Pinto-Plata et al., 2012).

We should also point out that several studies have found a relation between endothelial dysfunction and COPD (Cella et al., 2001; Moro et al., 2008; Nakanishi et al., 2011; Minet et al., 2012).

The relation between OSAS and cardiovascular disease involves a number of mechanisms such as the followings.

OSAS-associated disturbances, especially chronic intermittent hyopoxia and enhanced sympathetic activity, lead to up-regulation of the renin-angiotensin system and down-regulation of nitric oxide synthases (Fletcher et al., 1999; Prabhakar et al., 2001). When an obstructive apnea occurs, it is terminated by a sudden arousal, that is, lightening of sleep or awakening from sleep (Somers et al., 1995).

Furthermore, increased oxidative stress has been associated with development of cardiovascular diseases and can be promoted by the chronic intermittent hypoxia characteristic of OSAS (Park et al., 2007). In fact, a variety of studies suggest that oxidative stress is present in OSAS at levels relevant to tissues such as the arterial wall (Barcelo et al., 2006; Grebe et al., 2006). This process enhances lipid uptake into human macrophages and may contribute to atherosclerosis in OSAS patients (Lattimore et al., 2005).

Furthermore, OSAS decreases blood antioxidant status in high-BMI subjects and may change the relationship between oxidative stress markers (Wysocka et al., 2008).

Systemic inflammation is increasingly being recognized as a risk factor for a number of complications including atherosclerosis (Ross, 1999) and is a well-established factor in the pathogenesis of cardiovascular disease (Hansson, 2005). C-reactive protein is an important serum marker of inflammation with major implications for cardiovascular morbidity and atherogenesis (Rutter et al., 2004). C-reactive protein levels are increased in OSAS in accordance with disease severity (Shamsuzzaman et al., 2002; Kokturk et al., 2005; Punjabi & Beamer, 2007; Taheri et al., 2007).

A variety of findings support the existence of a relation between hypercoagulability, OSAS and cardiovascular disease. Patients with OSAS present higher plasma levels of several procoagulant factors such as fibrinogen (Reinhart et al., 2002; Tkacova et al., 2008), platelet activity (Akinnusi et al., 2009) and the fibrinolysis-inhibiting enzyme plasminogen activator inihibitor (PAI-1) (Von et al., 2006; Zamarron et al., 2008b).

Finally, a number of studies involving OSAS patients indicate an associated endothelial dysfunction (Nieto et al., 2004; Kohler et al., 2008; De la Peña et al., 2008). Endothelial dysfunction is frequently present in OSAS (Kheirandish-Gozal et al., 2010) and may have a potential role in the pathogenesis of vascular diseases that is pertinent to OSAS (Berger & Lavie, 2011). Several studies have reported higher endothelin-1 levels in OSAS patients (Phillips et al., 1999; Saarelainen & Hasan, 2000)

http://dx.doi.org/10.5772/57594

As inflammatory diseases, both OSAS and COPD are associated to higher cardiovascular risk. The mechanisms that may be involved different factors and include vascular inflammation, endothelial dysfunction, and tonic elevation of sympathetic neural activity (Figure 1).

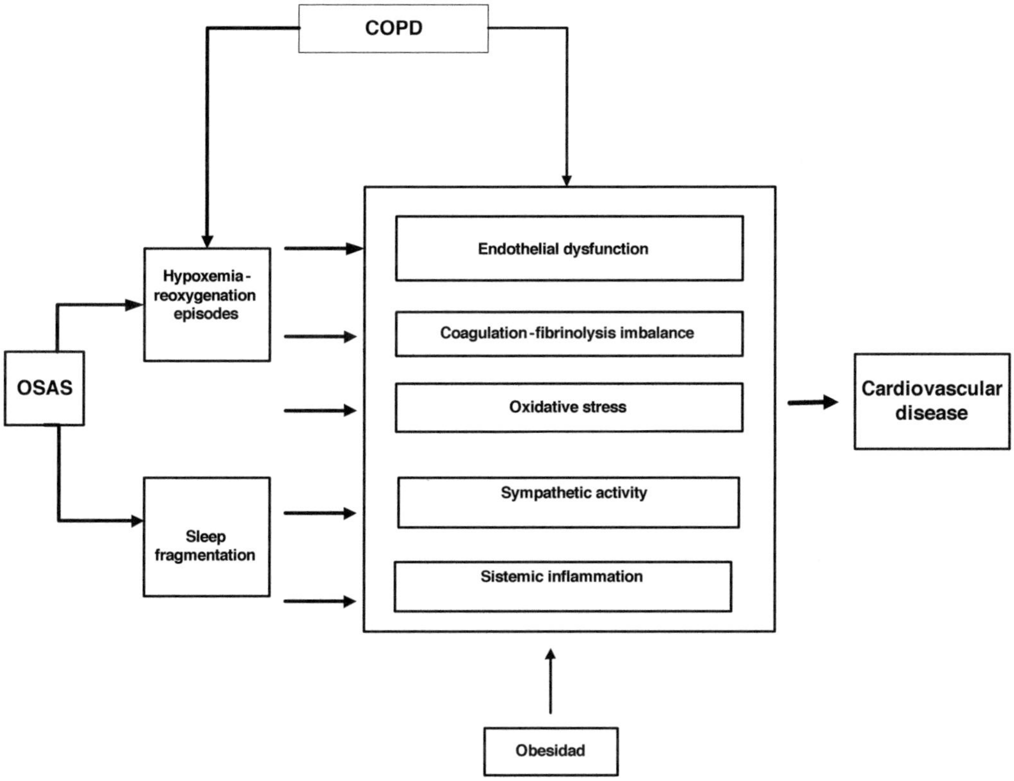

Figure 1. A schematic summary of the proposed sequence of events in obstructive sleep apnea syndrome (OSAS) and chronic obstructive pulmonary disease (COPD) starting from episodic hypoxia and sleep fragmentation

Evidence of systemic inflammation and oxidative stress in COPD and sleep apnea provides insight into potential interactions between both disorders that may predispose to cardiovascular disease (Lee & McNicholas, 2011). In sum, OSAS is one of the most frequent comorbidities and/or associations of COPD, and may bring on increased inflammation (Carratu & Resta, 2008; Macnee et al., 2008; Gilmartin et al., 2008; Shiina et al., 2012).

6. Clinical characteristics

The most common symptoms of OSAS patients include chronic loud snoring, excessive daytime sleepiness, personality changes, depression, impairment of thinking and deterioration of quality of life (Zamarron et al., 1998; Pichel et al., 2004). COPD patients, on the other hand, may present cough; sputum production; or dyspnea (Miravitlles et al., 2013).

Nevertheless, overlap patients present unique characteristics, which set them apart from either COPD-only or OSAS-only patients (Zamarron et al., 2008). After comparing overlap patients with OSAS-only patients, Radwan et al. found no significant differences in OSAS severity, mean arterial oxygen saturation during sleep, and BMI (Radwan et al., 1995). Chaouat et al. found that, compared to the OSAS-only group, the overlap population tended to be older, but similar BMI (Chaouat et al., 1995). O'Brien and Whitman found that overlap patients were older, and less obese than the OSAS-only group (O'Brien & Whitman, 2005). Resta el al. showed that overlap patients had higher $PaCO_2$ than OSAS-only group, but similar apnea hypopnea index. This author developed a model for predicting $PaCO_2$ in overlap patients based on PaO_2, FEV_1, and weight (Resta et al., 2002).

Cardiac arrhythmias and sudden death are common and important causes of mortality in patients with COPD (Yildiz et al 2002). Several factors such as hypoxemia, hypercapnia, acid-base disturbances, autonomic dysfunction, and medication may contribute to the development of arrhythmias in these patients (Sarubbi et al., 1997; Yildiz et al., 2002). Patients with OSAS have a higher frequency of cardiac rhythm disturbances and ST-segment depression episodes than snoring and control subjects. Moreover, ST-segment changes are related to sympathetic tone and sleep fragmentation, whereas most of the rhythm disturbances in OSAS patients are associated to sleep fragmentation, nocturnal hypoxemia, and sympathetic tone (Alonso-Fernandez et al., 2005).

Sleep disturbance in patients with COPD is usually related to nocturnal cough, wheezing, and shortness of breath (Weitzenblum & Chaouat, 2004). It is common for moderate to severe COPD patients to complain about poor-quality sleep, particularly elderly patients in the form of morning tiredness and early awakenings (Bellia et al., 2003). Sleep studies in COPD have shown frequent arousals and awakening, and decreased total sleep time with increased number of arousals (Fleetham et al., 1982). Furthermore, Sandek made reference to the fact that reduced average nocturnal oxygenation is associated with increased superficial sleep (Sandek et al., 1999).

In contrast, Sanders et al. observed that COPD patients without OSAS had minimally perturbed sleep. Thus, it appears that COPD per se does not affect or only slightly affects the quality of sleep. Instead, it may be that hypoxemia is a determinant of poor-quality sleep in patients with advanced COPD. In these patients, oxygen therapy has been shown to improve the quality of sleep, daytime hypoxemia and severe sleep-related oxygen desaturation (Sanders et al., 2003).

Colt indicates that in OSAS patients, one of the most incapacitating symptoms is excessive daytime somnolence, which results from disrupted sleep or nightime oxygen desaturation (Colt et al., 1991). In overlap patients, Sanders et al. observed that, compared to COPD-only subjects, they had higher Epworth sleepiness scores, lower total sleep time, lower sleep efficiency, and higher arousal index. Indeed, the quality of sleep in COPD seems to be influenced by the presence of OSAS but not by the severity of airway obstruction (Sanders et al., 2003).

Regarding hypercapnia, although overlap patients were expected to be at greater risk, Weitzenblum et al. found that diurnal pCO_2 levels were similar for COPD and overlap patients.

In fact, significant differences were only found with respect to healthy subjects (Weitzenblum et al., 2008).

In addition, some studies have shown that overlap syndrome has a major impact on quality of life. Mermigkis studied 30 subjects with overlap syndrome and 15 control subjects. Quality of life was determined by St George's Respiratory Questionnaire. The control group included subjects with COPD and no evidence of OSAS by polysomnography. All subjects were habitual snorers with normal Epworth Sleepiness Scale scores. Significant differences were found in total score and in each of the three questionnaire components suggesting worse quality of life in overlap patients. It is fair to say that OSAS has a major impact on quality of life in patients with overlap syndrome and can exist in COPD patients with habitual snoring even in the absence of daytime sleepiness (Mermigkis et al., 2007).

7. Diagnostic procedures

The diagnosis of OSAS should be based on clinical findings and confirmed by polysomnography which has traditionally been regarded as the gold standard for diagnosis (Kushida et al., 2005). However, alternatives that are less expensive and time-consuming are increasingly becoming popular (Flemons et al., 2003).

Subjects with COPD normally have well-preserved sleep architecture; hence, when faced with sleep complaints, the possible existence of associated sleep disorders should be considered and polysomnography applied for further characterization. Not all COPD patients necessarily need to be tested for OSAS. Nocturnal polysomnographic monitoring in COPD is usually performed when OSAS is suspected (Table 1). Only COPD subjects who have the typical risk factors for OSAS, such as obesity, chronic snoring, enlarged neck, daytime sleepiness, and hypertension, should be considered for further testing (Marrone et al., 2006; Lopez-Acevedo et al., 2009). Other indications include the presence of nocturnal hypoxaemia complications that are not explained by awake arterial oxygen levels, pulmonary hypertension, or cor pulmonale out of proportion to the severity of pulmonary function derangement in COPD patients whose daytime PaO2 is 60–65 mmHg (Douglas & Flenley, 1990).

Clinical suspicion of OSAS:	
	Headache upon awakening,
	Excessive daytime sleepiness.
	Snoring and breathing pauses
	Obesity
Normal daytime blood oxygen with	
	Cor pulmonale
	Polycithemia and normal daytime oxygen.

Table 1. Indications for nocturnal polysomnography in COPD

8. Treatment

Conventional oxygen therapy is prescribed to stable COPD patients who exhibit marked and persistent hypoxemia. This therapy is sufficient to correct even severe nocturnal desaturation and has favourable effects on the observed hypoxemia-related peaks in pulmonary hypertension (Boysen et al., 1979). Furthermore, some authors report that oxygen therapy improves the quality of sleep by shortening latency to sleep, increasing REM sleep as well as stages III and IV, and by decreasing number of arousals (Calverley et al., 1982).

All patients with OSAS should be counselled about the potential benefits of therapy and the risks of going without treatment as well as the value of avoiding factors that increase the severity of upper-airway obstruction, such as sleep deprivation; the use of alcohol, sedatives, and hypnotic agents; and excessive weight (Haynes, 2005). CPAP therapy is a well-established, widely used treatment (Giles et al., 2006), but, it is not suitable for all patients.

The coexistence of OSAS and COPD defines a high-risk group of patients because their awake and sleep related hypoxemia and hypoxemic cardiovascular consequences are more marked. Although the natural history of overlap syndrome is not well-known, a major aim of therapy should be to correct both upper airway obstructive episodes and sleep hypoxemia.

Treatment for overlap syndrome consists of CPAP or non-invasive positive pressure ventilation, with or without associated O2, for correction of the upper airway obstructive episodes and hypoxemia during sleep (Pronzato, 2010; Nural et al., 2013).

Sampol studied a group of overlap patients over three consecutive nights. This study found that the application of CPAP corrected apneas and hypopneas, but not oxygen desaturation. With the addition of oxygen at a flow of 1.5 L.min-1 at suboptimal CPAP levels, they observed an increase in apnea frequency, persistence of apneas at CPAP levels which eliminated them when no supplemental oxygen was administered, and longer duration of apneas and hypopneas. However, when the effective CPAP level was reached with supplemental oxygen, its efficacy in eliminating apneas and hypopneas was maintained and, furthermore, oxygen desaturation was corrected. The authors conclude that CPAP with supplemental oxygen constitutes a practical therapeutic alternative for hypoxic patients with overlap syndrome (Sampol et al., 1996).

De Miguel evaluated the effects of CPAP therapy on lung function in patients with overlap syndrome over two consecutive years. After six months of CPAP therapy, there were statistically significant increases in PaO_2, FEV_1, and FVC, accompanied by significant decreases in $PaCO_2$, serum bicarbonate levels, and alveolar-arterial oxygen difference. However, these patients also had significant weight loss during this time, which may explain the benefits observed. Also, the degree of obstruction, as reflected by the FEV_1/FVC ratio, did not change. Interestingly, there was no improvement from six to eighteen months, a period in which there were no changes in patient weight. Response of overlap syndrome patients to CPAP therapy was greater in the hypercapnic group, particularly in relation to improvement of arterial blood gases [13].

Mansfield and Naughton studied fourteen patients, ten of whom were able to tolerate CPAP for at least three months. They found an improvement in gas exchange and FEV_1 associated with a decrease in hospitalizations (Mansfield & Naughton, 1999). Similar results were reported by other studies (Peker et al., 1997;Marin et al., 2010).

CPAP treatment may have other potentially beneficial effects. Seeing as COPD is an inflammatory airways disorder and OSAS may act as an inflammatory stimulus, coexistent of both diseases in overlap may augment airway inflammation. Thus, the improvement in OSAS resulting from the application of CPAP may, in turn, lead to an improvement in the coexistent COPD. In some studies, the improvement in some markers of bronchial hyper responsiveness following the application of CPAP suggests the possibility that CPAP therapy may have a bronchodilator effect (Chan et al., 1988).

A decrease of serum C reactive protein in overlap patients following effective CPAP treatment shows that CPAP is an effective treatment method for systemic inflammation (Nural et al., 2013)

Nocturnal oxygen attenuates sleep desaturations among stable overlap patients and does not produce clinically significant increases in PaCO2. However, hypoxemia and hipercapnic may persist in the most severe overlap patients in spite of efficient application of nocturnal CPAP and oxygen therapy. For these patients, some authors recommend nocturnal treatment with positive pressure ventilators, and the monitoring of treatment effectiveness by sleep study (Marrone et al., 2006).

9. Prognosis

Regarding the complications that modify the natural history of COPD, it has previously been shown that, compared to COPD-only patients, overlap syndrome patients are at an increased risk for respiratory failure, pulmonary hypertension and cor pulmonale, independently of the degree of airway obstruction (Table 2).

Daytime pulmonary hypertension and right heart failure
High cardiovascular risk
Major impact on quality of life
Increased overall and cardiovascular mortality
Higher medical utilization and cost

Table 2. Overlap syndrome: impact of coexisting disease

In order to evaluate the cost-effectiveness of early interventions and disease management programs, Shaya studied the economic impact of OSAS among Medicaid beneficiaries with COPD. The diagnosis of concomitant COPD was associated with substantially higher medical utilization and cost than the diagnosis of either alone, and OSAS may add additional economic burden on beneficiaries who already have COPD or concomitant COPD (Shaya et al., 2009).

Machado carried out a prospective cohort study of 603 hypoxemic COPD patients receiving long-term oxygen therapy, 95 subjects were diagnosed with moderate-to-severe OSAS. After adjusting for several confounders, patients treated with CPAP had a significantly lower risk of death (Machado et al., 2009). This observational study indicated a positive effect of CPAP treatment on survival in moderate-to severe OSAS patients with hypoxemic COPD receiving long-term oxygen therapy. This study recommends an active search for OSAS in patients with hypoxemic COPD using a screening questionnaire and/or nocturnal oximetry.

Overlap syndrome exhibit both increased overall and cardiovascular mortality in patients with COPD. Marin et al. in a cohort of patients with SAS followed for nine years, patients with COPD and SAS had a relative risk of death of 1.79 (1.16 to 2.77), with cardiovascular and pulmonary causes the most common mortality even adjusted for the severity of COPD.

In conclusion, overlap syndrome constitutes a worsening of the complications inherent in either COPD or OSAS alone. Early identification and treatment of overlap syndrome is fundamental in order to avoid serious potential effects.

Author details

Carlos Zamarrón Sanz[1*], Carlos Rábade Castedo[1], Ester Zamarrón de Lucas[2], Emilio Morete Aracay[1] and Félix del Campo Matias[3]

*Address all correspondence to: carlos.zamarron.sanz@sergas.es

1 Servicio de Neumología, Hospital Clínico Universitario, Santiago, Spain

2 Hospital Universitario La Paz, Madrid, Spain

3 Hospital Universitario Rio Hortega, Universidad de Valladolid, Valladolid, Spain

References

[1] Agusti, A. G. (2005). COPD, a multicomponent disease: implications for management. *Respir.Med., 99,* 670-682.

[2] Akinnusi, M. E., Paasch, L. L., Szarpa, K. R., Wallace, P. K., & El Solh, A. A. (2009). Impact of nasal continuous positive airway pressure therapy on markers of platelet activation in patients with obstructive sleep apnea. *Respiration, 77,* 25-31.

[3] Alonso-Fernandez, A., Garcia-Rio, F., Racionero, M. A., Pino, J. M., Ortuno, F., Martinez, I. et al. (2005). Cardiac rhythm disturbances and ST-segment depression epi-

sodes in patients with obstructive sleep apnea-hypopnea syndrome and its mechanisms. *Chest, 127,* 15-22.

[4] Andreassen, H. & Vestbo, J. (2003). Chronic obstructive pulmonary disease as a systemic disease: an epidemiological perspective. *Eur.Respir.J.Suppl, 46,* 2s-4s.

[5] Ashutosh, K., Mead, G., & Dunsky, M. (1983). Early effects of oxygen administration and prognosis in chronic obstructive pulmonary disease and cor pulmonale. *Am.Rev.Respir.Dis., 127,* 399-404.

[6] Bady, E., Achkar, A., Pascal, S., Orvoen-Frija, E., & Laaban, J. P. (2000). Pulmonary arterial hypertension in patients with sleep apnoea syndrome. *Thorax, 55,* 934-939.

[7] Barcelo, A., Barbe, F., de la, P. M., Vila, M., Perez, G., Pierola, J. et al. (2006). Antioxidant status in patients with sleep apnoea and impact of continuous positive airway pressure treatment. *Eur.Respir.J., 27,* 756-760.

[8] Bednarek, M., Plywaczewski, R., Jonczak, L., & Zielinski, J. (2005). There is no relationship between chronic obstructive pulmonary disease and obstructive sleep apnea syndrome: a population study. *Respiration, 72,* 142-149.

[9] Bellia, V., Catalano, F., Scichilone, N., Incalzi, R. A., Spatafora, M., Vergani, C. et al. (2003). Sleep disorders in the elderly with and without chronic airflow obstruction: the SARA study. *Sleep, 26,* 318-323.

[10] Berger, S. & Lavie, L. (2011). Endothelial progenitor cells in cardiovascular disease and hypoxia-potential implications to obstructive sleep apnea. *Transl.Res., 158,* 1-13.

[11] Bonsignore, M. R., Marrone, O., Insalaco, G., & Bonsignore, G. (1994). The cardiovascular effects of obstructive sleep apnoeas: analysis of pathogenic mechanisms. *Eur.Respir.J., 7,* 786-805.

[12] Boysen, P. G., Block, A. J., Wynne, J. W., Hunt, L. A., & Flick, M. R. (1979). Nocturnal pulmonary hypertension in patients with chronic obstructive pulmonary disease. *Chest, 76,* 536-542.

[13] Bradley, T. D. & Phillipson, E. A. (1985). Pathogenesis and pathophysiology of the obstructive sleep apnea syndrome. *Med.Clin.North Am., 69,* 1169-1185.

[14] Calverley, P. M., Brezinova, V., Douglas, N. J., Catterall, J. R., & Flenley, D. C. (1982). The effect of oxygenation on sleep quality in chronic bronchitis and emphysema. *Am.Rev.Respir.Dis., 126,* 206-210.

[15] Carratu, P. & Resta, O. (2008). Is obstructive sleep apnoea a comorbidity of COPD and is it involved in chronic systemic inflammatory syndrome? *Eur.Respir.J., 31,* 1381-1382.

[16] Cella, G., Sbarai, A., Mazzaro, G., Vanzo, B., Romano, S., Hoppensteadt, T. et al. (2001). Plasma markers of endothelial dysfunction in chronic obstructive pulmonary disease. *Clin.Appl.Thromb.Hemost., 7,* 205-208.

[17] Chan, C. S., Woolcock, A. J., & Sullivan, C. E. (1988). Nocturnal asthma: role of snoring and obstructive sleep apnea. *Am.Rev.Respir.Dis., 137,* 1502-1504.

[18] Chaouat, A., Bugnet, A. S., Kadaoui, N., Schott, R., Enache, I., Ducolone, A. et al. (2005). Severe pulmonary hypertension and chronic obstructive pulmonary disease. *Am.J.Respir.Crit Care Med., 172,* 189-194.

[19] Chaouat, A., Weitzenblum, E., Krieger, J., Ifoundza, T., Oswald, M., & Kessler, R. (1995). Association of chronic obstructive pulmonary disease and sleep apnea syndrome. *Am.J.Respir.Crit Care Med., 151,* 82-86.

[20] Colt, H. G., Haas, H., & Rich, G. B. (1991). Hypoxemia vs sleep fragmentation as cause of excessive daytime sleepiness in obstructive sleep apnea. *Chest, 100,* 1542-1548.

[21] Curkendall, S. M., DeLuise, C., Jones, J. K., Lanes, S., Stang, M. R., Goehring E Jr et al. (2006). Cardiovascular disease in patients with chronic obstructive pulmonary disease, Saskatchewan Canada cardiovascular disease in COPD patients. *Ann.Epidemiol., 16,* 63-70.

[22] De la Peña, P. M., Barcelo, A., Barbe, F., Pierola, J., Pons, J., Rimbau, E. et al. (2008). Endothelial function and circulating endothelial progenitor cells in patients with sleep apnea syndrome. *Respiration, 76,* 28-32.

[23] De Lucas-Ramos, P., Izquierdo-Alonso, J. L., Rodriguez-Gonzalez Moro, J. M., Bellon-Cano, J. M., ncochea-Bermudez, J., Calle-Rubio, M. et al. (2008). [Cardiovascular risk factors in chronic obstructive pulmonary disease: results of the ARCE study]. *Arch.Bronconeumol., 44,* 233-238.

[24] De Lucas-Ramos, P., Izquierdo-Alonso, J. L., Rodriguez-Gonzalez Moro, J. M., Frances, J. F., Lozano, P. V., & Bellon-Cano, J. M. (2012). Chronic obstructive pulmonary disease as a cardiovascular risk factor. Results of a case-control study (CONSISTE study). *Int.J.Chron.Obstruct.Pulmon.Dis., 7,* 679-686.

[25] Doff, M. H., Hoekema, A., Wijkstra, P. J., van der Hoeven, J. H., Huddleston Slater, J. J., de Bont, L. G. et al. (2013). Oral appliance versus continuous positive airway pressure in obstructive sleep apnea syndrome: a 2-year follow-up. *Sleep, 36,* 1289-1296.

[26] Douglas, N. J. & Flenley, D. C. (1990). Breathing during sleep in patients with obstructive lung disease. *Am.Rev.Respir.Dis., 141,* 1055-1070.

[27] Douglas, N. J., White, D. P., Pickett, C. K., Weil, J. V., & Zwillich, C. W. (1982). Respiration during sleep in normal man. *Thorax, 37,* 840-844.

[28] Duran, J., Esnaola, S., Rubio, R., & Iztueta, A. (2001). Obstructive sleep apnea-hypopnea and related clinical features in a population-based sample of subjects aged 30 to 70 yr. *Am.J.Respir.Crit Care Med., 163,* 685-689.

[29] Fleetham, J., West, P., Mezon, B., Conway, W., Roth, T., & Kryger, M. (1982). Sleep, arousals, and oxygen desaturation in chronic obstructive pulmonary disease. The effect of oxygen therapy. *Am.Rev.Respir.Dis., 126,* 429-433.

[30] Flemons, W. W., Littner, M. R., Rowley, J. A., Gay, P., Anderson, W. M., Hudgel, D. W. et al. (2003). Home diagnosis of sleep apnea: a systematic review of the literature. An evidence review cosponsored by the American Academy of Sleep Medicine, the American College of Chest Physicians, and the American Thoracic Society. *Chest, 124,* 1543-1579.

[31] Flenley, D. C. (1985). Sleep in chronic obstructive lung disease. *Clin.Chest Med., 6,* 651-661.

[32] Fletcher, E. C., Schaaf, J. W., Miller, J., & Fletcher, J. G. (1987). Long-term cardiopulmonary sequelae in patients with sleep apnea and chronic lung disease. *Am.Rev.Respir.Dis., 135,* 525-533.

[33] Fletcher, E. C., Bao, G., & Li, R. (1999). Renin activity and blood pressure in response to chronic episodic hypoxia. *Hypertension, 34,* 309-314.

[34] Fuhrman, C., Jougla, E., Nicolau, J., Eilstein, D., & Delmas, M. C. (2006). Deaths from chronic obstructive pulmonary disease in France, 1979-2002: a multiple cause analysis. *Thorax, 61,* 930-934.

[35] Gan, W. Q., Man, S. F., Senthilselvan, A., & Sin, D. D. (2004). Association between chronic obstructive pulmonary disease and systemic inflammation: a systematic review and a meta-analysis. *Thorax, 59,* 574-580.

[36] Gastaut, H., Tassinari, C. A., & Duron, B. (1965). [Polygraphic study of diurnal and nocturnal (hypnic and respiratory) episodal manifestations of Pickwick syndrome]. *Rev.Neurol.(Paris), 112,* 568-579.

[37] Giles, T. L., Lasserson, T. J., Smith, B. J., White, J., Wright, J., & Cates, C. J. (2006). Continuous positive airways pressure for obstructive sleep apnoea in adults. *Cochrane.Database.Syst.Rev.,* CD001106.

[38] Gilmartin, G. S., Tamisier, R., Curley, M., & Weiss, J. W. (2008). Ventilatory, hemodynamic, sympathetic nervous system, and vascular reactivity changes after recurrent nocturnal sustained hypoxia in humans. *Am.J.Physiol Heart Circ.Physiol, 295,* H778-H785.

[39] Global Strategy for the Diagnosis, Management and Prevention of COPD, Global Initiative for Chronic Obstructive Lung Disease (GOLD) 2013. Available from http://www.goldcopd.org

[40] Grebe, M., Eisele, H. J., Weissmann, N., Schaefer, C., Tillmanns, H., Seeger, W. et al. (2006). Antioxidant vitamin C improves endothelial function in obstructive sleep apnea. *Am.J.Respir.Crit Care Med., 173,* 897-901.

[41] Guilleminault, C. (1985). Obstructive sleep apnea. The clinical syndrome and historical perspective. *Med.Clin.North Am., 69,* 1187-1203.

[42] Hansson, G. K. (2005). Inflammation, atherosclerosis, and coronary artery disease. *N.Engl.J.Med., 352,* 1685-1695.

[43] Hawrylkiewicz, I., Sliwinski, P., Gorecka, D., Plywaczewski, R., & Zielinski, J. (2004). Pulmonary haemodynamics in patients with OSAS or an overlap syndrome. *Monaldi Arch.Chest Dis., 61,* 148-152.

[44] Haynes, P. L. (2005). The role of behavioral sleep medicine in the assessment and treatment of sleep disordered breathing. *Clin.Psychol.Rev., 25,* 673-705.

[45] Hiestand, D. & Phillips, B. (2008). The overlap syndrome: chronic obstructive pulmonary disease and obstructive sleep apnea. *Crit Care Clin., 24,* 551-63, vii.

[46] Huiart, L., Ernst, P., & Suissa, S. (2005). Cardiovascular morbidity and mortality in COPD. *Chest, 128,* 2640-2646.

[47] Instituto Nacional de Estadística. Defunciones según la Causa de Muerte 2011. Available from :http://www.ine.es.

[48] Ioachimescu, O. C. & Teodorescu, M. (2013). Integrating the overlap of obstructive lung disease and obstructive sleep apnoea: OLDOSA syndrome. *Respirology.*, 18, 421-431.

[49] Izquierdo, J. L., Martinez, A., Guzman, E., de, L. P., & Rodriguez, J. M. (2010). Lack of association of ischemic heart disease with COPD when taking into account classical cardiovascular risk factors. *Int.J.Chron.Obstruct.Pulmon.Dis., 5,* 387-394.

[50] Izquierdo-Alonso, J. L., Rodriguez-Gonzalez Moro, J. M., de Lucas-Ramos, P., Unzueta, I., Ribera, X., Anton, E. et al. (2013). Prevalence and characteristics of three clinical phenotypes of chronic obstructive pulmonary disease (COPD). *Respir.Med., 107,* 724-731.

[51] Karadag, F., Kirdar, S., Karul, A. B., & Ceylan, E. (2008). The value of C-reactive protein as a marker of systemic inflammation in stable chronic obstructive pulmonary disease. *Eur.J.Intern.Med., 19,* 104-108.

[52] Kheirandish-Gozal, L., Bhattacharjee, R., Kim, J., Clair, H. B., & Gozal, D. (2010). Endothelial progenitor cells and vascular dysfunction in children with obstructive sleep apnea. *Am.J.Respir.Crit Care Med., 182,* 92-97.

[53] Kiely, J. L., Murphy, M., & McNicholas, W. T. (1999). Subjective efficacy of nasal CPAP therapy in obstructive sleep apnoea syndrome: a prospective controlled study. *Eur.Respir.J., 13,* 1086-1090.

[54] Kim, V., Han, M. K., Vance, G. B., Make, B. J., Newell, J. D., Hokanson, J. E. et al. (2011). The chronic bronchitic phenotype of COPD: an analysis of the COPDGene Study. *Chest, 140,* 626-633.

[55] Kohler, M., Craig, S., Nicoll, D., Leeson, P., Davies, R. J., & Stradling, J. R. (2008). Endothelial function and arterial stiffness in minimally symptomatic obstructive sleep apnea. *Am.J.Respir.Crit Care Med., 178,* 984-988.

[56] Kokturk, O., Ciftci, T. U., Mollarecep, E., & Ciftci, B. (2005). Elevated C-reactive protein levels and increased cardiovascular risk in patients with obstructive sleep apnea syndrome. *Int.Heart J., 46,* 801-809.

[57] Kushida, C. A., Littner, M. R., Morgenthaler, T., Alessi, C. A., Bailey, D., Coleman, J., Jr. et al. (2005). Practice parameters for the indications for polysomnography and related procedures: an update for 2005. *Sleep, 28,* 499-521.

[58] Kwon, J. S., Wolfe, L. F., Lu, B. S., & Kalhan, R. (2009). Hyperinflation is associated with lower sleep efficiency in COPD with co-existent obstructive sleep apnea. *COPD., 6,* 441-445.

[59] Lacedonia, D., Carpagnano, G. E., Aliani, M., Sabato, R., Foschino Barbaro, M. P., Spanevello, A. et al. (2013). Daytime PaO2 in OSAS, COPD and the combination of the two (overlap syndrome). *Respir.Med., 107,* 310-316.

[60] Lattimore, J. D., Wilcox, I., Nakhla, S., Langenfeld, M., Jessup, W., & Celermajer, D. S. (2005). Repetitive hypoxia increases lipid loading in human macrophages-a potentially atherogenic effect. *Atherosclerosis, 179,* 255-259.

[61] Lee, R. & McNicholas, W. T. (2011). Obstructive sleep apnea in chronic obstructive pulmonary disease patients. *Curr.Opin.Pulm.Med., 17,* 79-83.

[62] Lopez-Acevedo, M. N., Torres-Palacios, A., Elena Ocasio-Tascon, M., Campos-Santiago, Z., & Rodriguez-Cintron, W. (2009). Overlap syndrome: an indication for sleep studies? : A pilot study. *Sleep Breath.13, 409-413.*

[63] Lugaresi, E., Coccagna, G., Mantovani, M., & Lebrun, R. (1972). Some periodic phenomena arising during drowsiness and sleep in man. *Electroencephalogr.Clin.Neurophysiol., 32,* 701-705.

[64] Machado, M. C., Vollmer, W. M., Togeiro, S. M., Bilderback, A. L., Oliveira, M. V., Leitao, F. S. et al. (2009). CPAP treatment and survival of patients with moderate-to-severe OSAS and hypoxemic COPD. *Eur.Respir.J.* 35: 132-137

[65] Macnee, W., Maclay, J., & McAllister, D. (2008). Cardiovascular injury and repair in chronic obstructive pulmonary disease. *Proc.Am.Thorac.Soc., 5,* 824-833.

[66] Mansfield, D. & Naughton, M. T. (1999). Effects of continuous positive airway pressure on lung function in patients with chronic obstructive pulmonary disease and sleep disordered breathing. *Respirology., 4,* 365-370.

[67] Marin, J. M., Soriano, J. B., Carrizo, S. J., Boldova, A., & Celli, B. R. (2010). Outcomes in patients with chronic obstructive pulmonary disease and obstructive sleep apnea: the overlap syndrome. *Am.J.Respir.Crit Care Med., 182,* 325-331.

[68] Marrone, O., Salvaggio, A., & Insalaco, G. (2006). Respiratory disorders during sleep in chronic obstructive pulmonary disease. *Int.J.Chron.Obstruct.Pulmon.Dis., 1,* 363-372.

[69] McNicholas, W. T. (1997). Impact of sleep in respiratory failure. *Eur.Respir.J., 10,* 920-933.

[70] Mermigkis, C., Kopanakis, A., Foldvary-Schaefer, N., Golish, J., Polychronopoulos, V., Schiza, S. et al. (2007). Health-related quality of life in patients with obstructive sleep apnoea and chronic obstructive pulmonary disease (overlap syndrome). *Int.J.Clin.Pract., 61,* 207-211.

[71] Mills, N. L., Miller, J. J., Anand, A., Robinson, S. D., Frazer, G. A., Anderson, D. et al. (2008). Increased arterial stiffness in patients with chronic obstructive pulmonary disease: a mechanism for increased cardiovascular risk. *Thorax, 63,* 306-311.

[72] Minet, C., Vivodtzev, I., Tamisier, R., Arbib, F., Wuyam, B., Timsit, J. F. et al. (2012). Reduced six-minute walking distance, high fat-free-mass index and hypercapnia are associated with endothelial dysfunction in COPD. *Respir.Physiol Neurobiol., 183,* 128-134.

[73] Miravitlles, M., Soler-Cataluna, J. J., Calle, M., Molina, J., Almagro, P., Quintano, J. A. et al. (2013). A new approach to grading and treating COPD based on clinical phenotypes: summary of the Spanish COPD guidelines (GesEPOC). *Prim.Care Respir.J., 22,* 117-121.

[74] Moro, L., Pedone, C., Scarlata, S., Malafarina, V., Fimognari, F., & Antonelli-Inc (2008). Endothelial dysfunction in chronic obstructive pulmonary disease. *Angiology, 59,* 357-364.

[75] Nakanishi, K., Takeda, Y., Tetsumoto, S., Iwasaki, T., Tsujino, K., Kuhara, H. et al. (2011). Involvement of endothelial apoptosis underlying chronic obstructive pulmonary disease-like phenotype in adiponectin-null mice: implications for therapy. *Am.J.Respir.Crit Care Med., 183,* 1164-1175.

[76] Nieto, F. J., Herrington, D. M., Redline, S., Benjamin, E. J., & Robbins, J. A. (2004). Sleep apnea and markers of vascular endothelial function in a large community sample of older adults. *Am.J.Respir.Crit Care Med., 169,* 354-360.

[77] Nunomiya, K., Shibata, Y., Abe, S., Inoue, S., Igarashi, A., Yamauchi, K. et al. (2013). Hyperhomocysteinaemia predicts the decline in pulmonary function in healthy male smokers. *Eur.Respir.J., 42,* 18-27.

[78] Nural, S., Gunay, E., Halici, B., Celik, S., & Unlu, M. (2013). Inflammatory Processes and Effects of Continuous Positive Airway Pressure (CPAP) in Overlap Syndrome. *Inflammation, 36,* 66-74.

[79] O'Brien, A. & Whitman, K. (2005). Lack of benefit of continuous positive airway pressure on lung function in patients with overlap syndrome. *Lung, 183,* 389-404.

[80] Park, A. M., Nagase, H., Kumar, S. V., & Suzuki, Y. J. (2007). Effects of intermittent hypoxia on the heart. *Antioxid.Redox.Signal., 9,* 723-729.

[81] Peker, Y., Hedner, J., Johansson, A., & Bende, M. (1997). Reduced hospitalization with cardiovascular and pulmonary disease in obstructive sleep apnea patients on nasal CPAP treatment. *Sleep, 20,* 645-653.

[82] Phillips, B. G., Narkiewicz, K., Pesek, C. A., Haynes, W. G., Dyken, M. E., & Somers, V. K. (1999). Effects of obstructive sleep apnea on endothelin-1 and blood pressure. *J.Hypertens., 17,* 61-66.

[83] Pichel, F., Zamarron, C., Magan, F., del, C. F., varez-Sala, R., & Suarez, J. R. (2004). Health-related quality of life in patients with obstructive sleep apnea: effects of long-term positive airway pressure treatment. *Respir.Med., 98,* 968-976.

[84] Pinto-Plata, V. M., Mullerova, H., Toso, J. F., Feudjo-Tepie, M., Soriano, J. B., Vessey, R. S. et al. (2006). C-reactive protein in patients with COPD, control smokers and non-smokers. *Thorax, 61,* 23-28.

[85] Pinto-Plata, V., Casanova, C., Mullerova, H., de Torres, J. P., Corado, H., Varo, N. et al. (2012). Inflammatory and repair serum biomarker pattern: association to clinical outcomes in COPD. *Respir.Res., 13,* 71.

[86] Prabhakar, N. R., Fields, R. D., Baker, T., & Fletcher, E. C. (2001). Intermittent hypoxia: cell to system. *Am.J.Physiol Lung Cell Mol.Physiol, 281,* L524-L528.

[87] Pronzato, C. (2010). Chronic obstructive pulmonary disease and obstructive sleep apnea. Association, consequences and treatment. *Monaldi Arch.Chest Dis., 73,* 155-161.

[88] Punjabi, N. M. & Beamer, B. A. (2007). C-reactive protein is associated with sleep disordered breathing independent of adiposity. *Sleep, 30,* 29-34.

[89] Rabe, K. F., Hurd, S., Anzueto, A., Barnes, P. J., Buist, S. A., Calverley, P. et al. (2007). Global strategy for the diagnosis, management, and prevention of chronic obstructive pulmonary disease: GOLD executive summary. *Am.J.Respir.Crit Care Med., 176,* 532-555.

[90] Radwan, L., Maszczyk, Z., Koziorowski, A., Koziej, M., Cieslicki, J., Sliwinski, P. et al. (1995a). Control of breathing in obstructive sleep apnoea and in patients with the overlap syndrome. *Eur.Respir.J., 8,* 542-545.

[91] Reinhart, W. H., Oswald, J., Walter, R., & Kuhn, M. (2002). Blood viscosity and platelet function in patients with obstructive sleep apnea syndrome treated with nasal continuous positive airway pressure. *Clin.Hemorheol.Microcirc., 27,* 201-207.

[92] Remmers, J. E., deGroot, W. J., Sauerland, E. K., & Anch, A. M. (1978). Pathogenesis of upper airway occlusion during sleep. *J.Appl.Physiol, 44,* 931-938.

[93] Resta, O., Foschino Barbaro, M. P., Brindicci, C., Nocerino, M. C., Caratozzolo, G., & Carbonara, M. (2002). Hypercapnia in overlap syndrome: possible determinant factors. *Sleep Breath., 6,* 11-18.

[94] Ross, R. (1999). Atherosclerosis--an inflammatory disease. *N.Engl.J.Med., 340,* 115-126.

[95] Rutter, M. K., Meigs, J. B., Sullivan, L. M., D'Agostino, R. B., Sr., & Wilson, P. W. (2004). C-reactive protein, the metabolic syndrome, and prediction of cardiovascular events in the Framingham Offspring Study. *Circulation, 110,* 380-385.

[96] Saarelainen, S. & Hasan, J. (2000). Circulating endothelin-1 and obstructive sleep apnoea. *Eur.Respir.J., 16,* 794-795.

[97] Sampol, G., Sagales, M. T., Roca, A., de, l. C., Bofill, J. M., & Morell, F. (1996). Nasal continuous positive airway pressure with supplemental oxygen in coexistent sleep apnoea-hypopnoea syndrome and severe chronic obstructive pulmonary disease. *Eur.Respir.J., 9,* 111-116.

[98] Sandek, K., Andersson, T., Bratel, T., Hellstrom, G., & Lagerstrand, L. (1999). Sleep quality, carbon dioxide responsiveness and hypoxaemic patterns in nocturnal hypoxaemia due to chronic obstructive pulmonary disease (COPD) without daytime hypoxaemia. *Respir.Med., 93,* 79-87.

[99] Sanders, M. H., Newman, A. B., Haggerty, C. L., Redline, S., Lebowitz, M., Samet, J. et al. (2003). Sleep and sleep-disordered breathing in adults with predominantly mild obstructive airway disease. *Am.J.Respir.Crit Care Med., 167,* 7-14.

[100] Sarubbi, B., Esposito, V., Ducceschi, V., Meoli, I., Grella, E., Santangelo, L. et al. (1997). Effect of blood gas derangement on QTc dispersion in severe chronic obstructive pulmonary disease: evidence of an electropathy? *Int.J.Cardiol., 58,* 287-292.

[101] Schunemann, H. J., Dorn, J., Grant, B. J., Winkelstein, W., Jr., & Trevisan, M. (2000). Pulmonary function is a long-term predictor of mortality in the general population: 29-year follow-up of the Buffalo Health Study. *Chest, 118,* 656-664.

[102] Seemungal, T. A., Lun, J. C., Davis, G., Neblett, C., Chinyepi, N., Dookhan, C. et al. (2007). Plasma homocysteine is elevated in COPD patients and is related to COPD severity. *Int.J.Chron.Obstruct.Pulmon.Dis., 2,* 313-321.

[103] Shamsuzzaman, A. S., Winnicki, M., Lanfranchi, P., Wolk, R., Kara, T., Accurso, V. et al. (2002). Elevated C-reactive protein in patients with obstructive sleep apnea. *Circulation, 105,* 2462-2464.

[104] Shaya, F. T., Lin, P. J., Aljawadi, M. H., & Scharf, S. M. (2009). Elevated economic burden in obstructive lung disease patients with concomitant sleep apnea syndrome. *Sleep Breath, 13: 317-323.*

[105] Shiina, K., Tomiyama, H., Takata, Y., Yoshida, M., Kato, K., Nishihata, Y. et al. (2012). Overlap syndrome: additive effects of COPD on the cardiovascular damages in patients with OSA. *Respir.Med., 106,* 1335-1341.

[106] Sobradillo, V., Miravitlles, M., Jimenez, C. A., Gabriel, R., Viejo, J. L., Masa, J. F. et al. (1999). [Epidemiological study of chronic obstructive pulmonary disease in Spain (IBERPOC): prevalence of chronic respiratory symptoms and airflow limitation]. *Arch.Bronconeumol., 35,* 159-166.

[107] Somers, V. K., Dyken, M. E., Clary, M. P., & Abboud, F. M. (1995). Sympathetic neural mechanisms in obstructive sleep apnea. *J.Clin.Invest, 96,* 1897-1904.

[108] Taheri, S., Austin, D., Lin, L., Nieto, F. J., Young, T., & Mignot, E. (2007). Correlates of serum C-reactive protein (CRP)--no association with sleep duration or sleep disordered breathing. *Sleep, 30,* 991-996.

[109] Takabatake, N., Nakamura, H., Abe, S., Inoue, S., Hino, T., Saito, H. et al. (2000). The relationship between chronic hypoxemia and activation of the tumor necrosis factor-alpha system in patients with chronic obstructive pulmonary disease. *Am.J.Respir.Crit Care Med., 161,* 1179-1184.

[110] Tkacova, R., Dorkova, Z., Molcanyiova, A., Radikova, Z., Klimes, I., & Tkac, I. (2008). Cardiovascular risk and insulin resistance in patients with obstructive sleep apnea. *Med.Sci.Monit., 14,* CR438-CR444.

[111] Tuncel, U., Inancli, H. M., Kurkcuoglu, S. S., & Enoz, M. (2012). A comparison of unilevel and multilevel surgery in obstructive sleep apnea syndrome. *Ear Nose Throat J., 91,* E13-E18.

[112] Von, K. R., Loredo, J. S., ncoli-Israel, S., & Dimsdale, J. E. (2006). Association between sleep apnea severity and blood coagulability: Treatment effects of nasal continuous positive airway pressure. *Sleep Breath., 10,* 139-146.

[113] Weitzenblum, E., Krieger, J., Apprill, M., Vallee, E., Ehrhart, M., Ratomaharo, J. et al. (1988). Daytime pulmonary hypertension in patients with obstructive sleep apnea syndrome. *Am.Rev.Respir.Dis., 138,* 345-349.

[114] Weitzenblum, E. & Chaouat, A. (2004). Sleep and chronic obstructive pulmonary disease. *Sleep Med.Rev., 8,* 281-294.

[115] Weitzenblum, E., Chaouat, A., Kessler, R., & Canuet, M. (2008). Overlap syndrome: obstructive sleep apnea in patients with chronic obstructive pulmonary disease. *Proc.Am.Thorac.Soc., 5,* 237-241.

[116] White, D. P., Weil, J. V., & Zwillich, C. W. (1985). Metabolic rate and breathing during sleep. *J.Appl.Physiol, 59,* 384-391.

[117] Wysocka, E., Cofta, S., Cymerys, M., Gozdzik, J., Torlinski, L., & Batura-Gabryel, H. (2008). The impact of the sleep apnea syndrome on oxidant-antioxidant balance in the blood of overweight and obese patients. *J.Physiol Pharmacol., 59 Suppl 6,* 761-769.

[118] Yildiz, P., Tukek, T., Akkaya, V., Sozen, A. B., Yildiz, A., Korkut, F. et al. (2002). Ventricular arrhythmias in patients with COPD are associated with QT dispersion. *Chest, 122,* 2055-2061.

[119] Young, T., Palta, M., Dempsey, J., Skatrud, J., Weber, S., & Badr, S. (1993). The occurrence of sleep-disordered breathing among middle-aged adults. *N.Engl.J.Med., 328,* 1230-1235.

[120] Zamarron, C., Garcia, P., V, Morete, E., & del Campo, M. F. (2008). Association of chronic obstructive pulmonary disease and obstructive sleep apnea consequences. *Int.J.Chron.Obstruct.Pulmon.Dis., 3,* 671-682.

[121] Zamarron, C., Gude, F., Otero, Y., Alvarez, J. M., Golpe, A., & Rodriguez, J. R. (1999). Prevalence of sleep disordered breathing and sleep apnea in 50- to 70-year-old individuals. A survey. *Respiration, 66,* 317-322.

[122] Zamarron, C., Gude, F., Otero, Y.,Alvarez Dobaño, J. M., Golpe, A., & Rodriguez, S., Jr. (1998). [Symptoms of sleep apnea syndrome in the general population]. Arch.Bronconeumol., 34, 245-249.

[123] Zamarron, C., Ricoy, J., Riveiro, A., & Gude, F. (2008). Plasminogen activator inhibitor-1 in obstructive sleep apnea patients with and without hypertension. Lung, 186, 151-156.

Chapter 7

Contribution of Autonomic Nervous System to the Hypertension Induced by Obstructive Sleep Apnea

Rodrigo Iturriaga and Juan Idiaquez

Additional information is available at the end of the chapter

http://dx.doi.org/10.5772/57565

1. Introduction

Cardiovascular diseases are the leading cause of morbidity and mortality in the adult population. The most common risk condition to almost all cardiovascular diseases is hypertension. The obstructive sleep apnea (OSA) syndrome, a growing worldwide sleep-breathing disorder is recognized as an independent risk factor for hypertension and is associated with other cardiovascular diseases, such as stroke, pulmonary hypertension, coronary artery disease and stroke. OSA is characterized by repeated episodes of airflow detention during sleep produced by the upper airway collapse. Among the disturbances produced by OSA, the chronic intermittent hypoxia is considered the main factor for the progression of the systemic hypertension. Although the link between OSA and systemic hypertension is well established, the pathogenic mechanisms responsible for the hypertension are not entirely understood. Autonomic dysfunction, oxidative stress and inflammation have been proposed as potential hypertensive mechanisms. However, conclusions from studies in OSA patients are controversial, because of concomitant comorbidities (i.e. obesity, metabolic disorders and cardiovascular diseases), which are confounding factors that increases the cardiovascular risk associated with OSA. Thus, experimental models of rodents exposed to chronic intermittent hypoxia, which reproduced several pathologic cardiovascular features of OSA, are the gold-standard to study the pathogenic mechanisms involved in the OSA-induced hypertension. In this chapter, we will review and discuss the evidence supporting an essential role of the carotid body chemoreceptor and the contribution of the autonomic nervous system to the progression of the hypertension in OSA patients and animals exposed to chronic intermittent hypoxia.

2. Pathogenic mechanisms of the hypertension induced by OSA

The OSA syndrome elicited by repeated airflow total or partial occlusions is diagnosed when patients has an apnea-hypopnea index (AHI) > 10 events/hour. OSA affects up to 9% of the adults men and 4% of women worldwide population [111]. However, according to a report of the American Heart Association in collaboration with the National Center on Sleep Disorders Research, "85% of patients with clinically significant and treatable OSA have never been diagnosed, and referral populations of OSA patients represent only the *tip of the iceberg* of OSA prevalence". Therefore, the estimated adult population that present an AHI of 5 is ~20% [100]. The OSA syndrome is associated with clinical neurobehavioral dysfunction, such as daytime sleepiness, fatigue, depressed mood, attention and executive deficits, and verbal and visual-spatial memory impairments [5, 67]. Nevertheless, the OSA syndrome is also associated with diurnal systemic hypertension (~50% of the OSA patients developed systemic hypertension), and with stroke, pulmonary hypertension, coronary artery disease and atrial fibrillation [3, 8, 12, 19; 28, 30, 35, 52, 53, 64, 74, 79, 100].

Several epidemiological studies have shown that OSA is an independent risk factor for the progression of the hypertension. Indeed, OSA patients show a positive relationship between AHI and the hypertension, which is independent of other risks [23, 60, 61, 85, 96, 100, 111, 112]. Moreover, results obtained from the Wisconsin Sleep Cohort (an ongoing 21-years longitudinal study performed on 1500 Wisconsin state employees) have shown that untreated OSA patients have a high mortality risk associated with AHI [74, 112].

Although the link between OSA and hypertension is well established, the mechanisms underlying the hypertension are not entirely known. The most accepted explanation proposes that chronic intermittent hypoxia produces oxidative stress, inflammation, and sympathetic hyperactivity, which led to endothelial dysfunction and hypertension [19, 25, 28, 41, 43, 52, 53, 65, 99, 100], but it is likely that intrathoracic pressure changes causing excessive mechanical stress on large artery walls and the heart, and arousal-induced sympathetic hyperactivity may also contribute to the endothelial dysfunction [47]. OSA is characterized by repeated episodes of total or partial airflow detention during sleep produced by the pharyngeal collapse, eliciting intermittent hypoxia and hypercapnia, negative intrathoraxic pressure, sleep fragmentation and arousal. During the airflow occlusion, the resulting hypoxia and hypercapnia stimulates the carotid body chemoreceptors producing reflex ventilatory, sympathetic and hypertensive responses. Among these disturbances, the chronic intermittent hypoxia is considered the main factor for the development of the hypertension [1, 19, 33, 41, 43, 51, 55, 56, 82, 83, 88, 93, 100]. However, conclusions from studies performed in OSA patients are partial and somehow controversial, because invasive procedures are precluded because of ethical reasons in humans, and OSA patients often present concomitant morbidities (i.e. obesity, metabolic alterations and other cardiovascular diseases), which are confounding factors that increase the cardiovascular risk. Therefore, experimental models of rodents exposed to intermittent hypoxia, which simulates the hypoxic-reoxygenation cycles and reproduce several of the cardiovascular pathologic features of OSA including hypertension, are the gold-standard to study the pathogenic mechanisms involved in progression of the cardiovascular and respiratory alterations induced by OSA [15-18, 22, 27, 43, 83-84, 86, 88, 95].

3. Clinical aspects of OSA

There are a strong association between OSA and systemic hypertension in human patients. Indeed, several studies have shown that the prevalence of OSA is higher in hypertensive patients, while other studies have shown that OSA increases the predisposition for hypertension. In addition, there are observational studies that showed that patients with hypertension presented a high incidence of OSA, some of these studies are cross-sectional (27, 46, 51, 109]. It has been found in patients with resistant hypertension, that the main secondary cause was OSA [81]. On other hand, cross-sectional studies have shown that patients with sleep breathing disorders, including OSA and snoring, present a strong correlation with hypertension [8, 74, 112]. Prospective studies also showed a strong association between AHI and THE increased arterial blood pressure [85]. It is relevant to note that the OSA-hypertension link is independent from other comorbidities like obesity [33, 45, 51, 79, 100]. Other study performed in OSA patients without hypertension, which were follow-up during five years for the risk of hypertension, concluded that there is a trend of association between AHI > 30 and the occurrence of the hypertension [75]. OSA patients without treatment presented high risk of hypertension than those patients treated with continuous positive airway pressure (CPAP) therapy [61].

OSA and hypertensive patients frequently present a combination of comorbidities including obesity, diabetes and cardiovascular diseases ([1, 33, 45, 54, 56, 64, 100]. The mechanisms that could explain the association between OSA and hypertension are still in ongoing research. As was mentioned before, the pathogenesis of the association between OSA and hypertension is likely to be multifactorial, involving a varied range of pathogenic mechanisms comprising a group of systemic factors including inflammation, oxidative stress and metabolic dysregulation, which are beyond the scope of this review. Evidence supporting the role played by sympathetic dysfunction has been demonstrated by different invasive and noninvasive methods that quantify sympathetic activity in patients with OSA, the main methods reported are:

3.1. Muscle sympathetic nerve activity in OSA patients

This technique is based on the microneurographic recording with a tungsten electrode of the muscle sympathetic nerve activity in the peroneal nerve, which produce vasoconstriction in blood vessel of skeletal muscles. The muscle sympathetic nerve discharge plays a fundamental role in the homeostasis of the systemic arterial blood pressure. Studies comparing muscle sympathetic discharges between OSA patients and controls showed that patients had higher basal levels of muscle sympathetic nerve discharges [71-73, 99]. Also intermittent hypoxia in humans produced hypertension and elevated the muscle sympathetic nerve discharges [29]. Continuous positive air pressure therapy decrease muscle sympathetic nerve discharges overactivity in OSA patients [39, 72, 73, 99].

3.2. Heart rate variability in OSA patients

The spectral analysis of heart rate variability has two major components defined as the low frequency (LF) band related to sympathetic influences, and the high frequency (HF) band related mainly to vagal influences and respiratory sinus arrhythmia. The LF/HF ratio is believed to be an index of the sympathovagal balance on heart rate [105]. Normotensive patients with recently diagnosed OSA showed a shift of the HRV spectral indexes towards the low frequency band, which is associated with increased sympathetic discharges in the peroneal nerve [70, 97]. The spectral analysis of heart rate variability is performed using a Fast Fourier Transform or autoregressive methods. The spectrum of R-R intervals is assess using the following frequency bands: very low frequency: DC-0.04 Hz, low frequency (LF): 0.04-0.15 Hz and high frequency (HF): 0.15-0.4 Hz in the frequency domain. HF power reflects the activity of parasympathetic nervous system activity, whereas LF power reflects a combination of sympathetic and parasympathetic activity [92, 105]. OSA patients showed increased sympathetic and reduced vagal modulation of HRV in comparison with controls [2, 4]. This symphato-vagal imbalance is modified with CPAP therapy; in OSA patients with hypertension CPAP administration reduced the LF power [11, 114].

3.3. Catecholamine measurements in OSA patients

The measurement of blood or urinary catecholamines gives information about their release from neurons and from the adrenal medulla. Baseline values of the plasmatic concentration of norepinephrine (NE) characterize the balance between the amount of NE released and then re-uptake into the nerve terminals. The urinary NE is the amount of NE that is being eliminated by excretion and metabolism. Plasmatic concentration of epinephrine (E) represents a balance between adreno-medullary release, excretion and metabolism. In OSA patients, studies of catecholamines concentrations had shown the presence of elevated levels of catecholamines in plasma and urine [62, 24, 113], suggesting and elevated sympathetic activity. OSA patients with elevated NE levels in plasma and urine showed severe hypertension and excessive sweating, similar to what happened in pheochromocytoma, improved their condition with CPAP therapy ([36]. It has also been shown that CPAP reduces NE levels in patients with severe OSA [101, 113, 114]. In children with OSA an association between AHI and urinary NE and E has been also reported [76].

3.4. Noninvasive cardiovascular autonomic tests in OSA patients

These tests are grouping in two main categories: sympathetic and cardiovagal tests. The sympathetic tests include arterial blood pressure response to gravitational stress, isometric exercise and cold stimuli. Cardiovagal autonomic tests include heart rate changes on deep breathing, Valsalva maneuver ratio and heart rate changes on standing. These tests are performed during wakefulness and they have shown a diurnal sympathetic dysfunction [6, 14, 66, 103]. Also parasympathetic cardiac dysfunction has been found in OSA patients [14, 66, 107].Overall, the results of these tests suggest an increased sympathetic tone and a decreased parasympathetic cardiac function in OSA patients.

http://dx.doi.org/10.5772/57565

4. Autonomic dysfunction in animals exposed to chronic intermittent hypoxia

Patients recently diagnosed with OSA, show enhanced vasopressor and ventilatory responses to acute hypoxia [69, 71], sympathetic hyperactivity, demonstrated by an increased muscle sympathetic neural activity [9, 68, 72-73, 99] and a higher accumulation of 24-h urinary norepinephrine [21]. Similarly, animals exposed to chronic intermittent hypoxia present enhanced sympathetic discharges and respiratory responses to acute hypoxia, and develop systemic hypertension [15, 20, 25, 26, 34, 37, 48, 59, 86, 87, 92, 115]. The autonomic alteration is characterized by an enhanced sympathetic outflow, reduction of the efficiency of the baroreflexes sensitivity and alterations of heart rate variability. Indeed, non-invasive spectral analysis of heart rate variability suggested a preponderance of the sympathetic drive in animals exposed to chronic intermittent hypoxia [15, 20, 57, 86, 88, 92], similarly to what was observed patients with OSA [68,72, 97,99]. Thus, it is likely that the enhanced sympathetic activity along with the reduction of the baroreflex sensitivity could impair heart rate variability and the regulation of vasomotor tone of blood vessels contributing to the hypertension. In addition, chronic intermittent hypoxia elicits vagal withdrawal, attributed in part to neuronal loss in ambiguous nucleus [57, 110].

Using a protocol of short hypoxic cycles (10% O_2, 10 times/hr for 8 hrs), we found that exposure of cats to chronic intermittent hypoxia for 4 days enhanced the ventilatory responses induced by acute hypoxia and reduced the sensitivity of the baroreflex control of heart rate, but did not evoke hypertension or enhanced the vasopressor responses to hypoxia [88, 90, 92]. However, normotensive animals exposed to chronic intermittent hypoxia like normotensive OSA patients, show a similar increased LF/HF ratio [88, 92]. Besides that, we found a positive linear correlation (r=0.97) between the LH/HF ratio and the baseline carotid body chemosensory discharges in the hypoxic-treated cats, suggesting that the potentiation of carotid body chemosensory discharges may be linked to early changes in the autonomic control of heart rate in cats exposed to short-term chronic intermittent hypoxia [92]. Thus, our results suggest that the hypertension induced by chronic intermittent hypoxia is preceded by early alterations in the autonomic balance of the heart rate, associated with an enhanced carotid body chemosensory response to hypoxia and a decreased baroreflex control [88, 92]. Lai et al., [See in 49] also found that chronic intermittent hypoxia increases the LF component and the LF/HF ratio of the blood pressure variability before the onset of the hypertension in conscious rats exposed to intermittent hypoxia.

5. Contribution of the carotid body to the cardiorespiratory alterations in OSA patients and animals exposed to chronic intermittent hypoxia

The enhanced cardiorespiratory responses to acute hypoxia observed in OSA patients has been attributed to a potentiated hypoxic peripheral chemoreflexes [12, 58, 69, 71], suggesting that carotid body chemoreceptors play a main role in the pathological alterations induced by OSA.

Moreover, Fletcher et al., [See in 26] found that the bilateral carotid body denervation prevented the hypertension in rats exposed to chronic intermittent hypoxia, suggesting that the carotid body contributes to the cardiovascular pathologies induced by OSA. In the last years, the proposal that the carotid body is involved in the progression of the intermittent hypoxia-induced hypertension received substantial attention [19, 22, 25, 28, 41, 43, 98, 100].

A growing body of new evidence supports the proposal that the carotid body is involved in the generation of the hypertension in OSA patients and animals exposed to intermittent hypoxia. OSA patients present enhanced ventilatory, pressor and sympathetic responses to acute hypoxia, attributed to a potentiation of the peripheral hypoxic chemoreflexes [58, 100]. Narkiewicz et al. [See in 69, 71] studied the reflex ventilatory, tachycardic and vasopressor responses to acute hypoxia in untreated normotensive patients with OSA, and found that the hypoxic stimulation produce larger increases in volume-minute ventilation, heart rate and arterial blood pressure in OSA patients than control subjects. Thus, the available data support the idea that the enhanced chemoreflex response observed in OSA patients is produced by the intermittent hypoxia. Similarly, animals exposed to chronic intermittent hypoxia show enhanced hypoxic ventilatory responses to acute hypoxia [15, 18, 43, 44, 87] and long-term facilitation of respiratory motor responses [63, 83, 88]. Recording of chemosensory nerve impulses from the carotid sinus nerve have confirmed the idea that chronic intermittent hypoxia produces long-term facilitation of the carotid body chemosensory responses to hypoxia. Indeed, exposure of rats and cats to intermittent hypoxia for few days increases the basal carotid body discharges measured in normoxia and enhances the chemosensory responses to acute hypoxia [15, 18, 43, 82-84, 88, 90].

The carotid body, located in the bifurcations of the carotid arteries is the main arterial oxygen chemoreceptor in terms of its contribution to the ventilatory reflex responses. In mammals, the hypoxic stimulation of the carotid body increases the sympathetic discharges to the arterial blood vessels and heart, producing hypertension. The primary oxygen sensors in the carotid body are the glomus cells, which are in synaptic contact with the nerve terminals of the chemosensory petrosal neurons [31, 40, 42]. The current model of chemoreception states that hypoxia induces the inhibition of voltage-independent tandem pore domain potassium channels (TASK K^+), leading to the depolarization of the glomus cells, the entry of Ca^{2+}through L-type Ca^{2+}channels, and the subsequent release of excitatory transmitters (Acetylcholine and adenosine triphosphate), which increases the discharges of the nerve endings of the petrosal chemosensory neurons [40, 42]. Recently, we found that chronic intermittent hypoxia potentiates the hypoxic inhibition of the TASK-like K^+channel currents in glomus cells from intermittent hypoxia rats. This novel effect of intermittent hypoxia may contribute to explain its enhancing effect on carotid body hypoxic chemoreception [77]. The carotid body is a polymodal chemosensory receptor, which is activated by hypoxia, hypercapnia, acidosis, stop flow, temperature and respond to the levels of glucose [31]. The carotid body has been involved in several sympathetic-mediated diseases such as hypertension, heart failure, diabetes and renal failure [94]. Moreover, the denervation or ablation of the carotid body has been proposed for the treatment of severe and resistant hypertension [78].

6. Mediators of enhanced carotid body chemosensory responses to hypoxia in animal models of OSA

Reactive oxygen species (ROS) and reactive nitrogen species (RNS), and pro-inflammatory agents have been proposed as mediators of cardiovascular and cognitive alterations in OSA patients [7, 13, 33, 45, 52, 65, 102] and animal models [10, 15-18, 44, 48, 82, 84, 106]. Studies performed in OSA patients and animals exposed to intermittent hypoxia showed that the hypoxia-reoxygenation episodes produce systemic oxidative stress due to the accumulation of ROS and RNS, which are potential sources of cellular damage. Recently, we tested the hypothesis that oxidative stress contributes to the carotid body chemosensory potentiation and the progression of the hypertension in rats exposed to chronic intermittent hypoxia [15, 18, 44]. We found that intermittent hypoxia increased the plasma lipid peroxidation and the formation of the oxidative stress marker 3-nitrotyrosine in the carotid body. In addition, chronic intermittent hypoxia enhances carotid body chemosensory and reflex ventilatory responses to hypoxia, alters hear rate variability and elicits hypertension [15]. Ascorbic acid treatment reduced the increased systemic and local carotid body oxidative stress, the potentiation of the carotid body chemosensory and ventilatory responses to hypoxia, as well as the hypertension [15]. These results agree and extend previous observations that antioxidant pre-treatment prevented the carotid body chemosensory potentiation [80, 82] and the hypertension [106] in rats exposed to intermittent hypoxia. Although, these results strongly suggest that the carotid body chemosensory potentiation is mediated by oxidative stress [15, 43, 44, 80], it is matter of debate if ROS *perse* increases the carotid body chemosensory discharges [32]. Thus, it is likely that other molecule downstream the ROS signals mediate the effects of ROS on carotid body chemoreception induced by intermittent hypoxia. The CB, the main contributor to the sympathetic activation and hypertension following intermittent hypoxia is extremely sensitive to peroxynitrites formation [15] Thus, RNS formation is a common feature in both human and experimental OSA models, suggesting that may participate in the OSA pathophysiology. In conclusion, the available evidence supports and extends the idea that both oxidative and nitrosative stress plays a pivotal role in OSA pathophysiology.

Among the molecules upregulated in the carotid body by intermittent hypoxia, such as endotelin-1 (ET-1), vascular endothelial growth factor (VEGF), and inducible nitric oxide synthase (iNOS) [15-18, 50, 89-91], pro-inflammatory cytokines have been proposed as mediators of the carotid body chemosensory potentiation induced by intermittent hypoxia [16, 18, 43, 44, 50] and cardiovascular pathologies in OSA patients [7, 65, 108, 104]. We found that chronic intermittent hypoxia induced a ROS-dependent increases of tumor necrosis factor (TNF) and Interleukin 1β (IL-1β) in the carotid body, suggesting that these pro-inflammatory cytokines may mediate the ROS-induced carotid body potentiation [16, 18]. To test this hypothesis, we studied the effects of ibuprofen on the increased TNF-α and IL-1β levels in the rat carotid body, the potentiation of carotid body chemosensory and ventilatory hypoxic responses and the hypertension [18]. Ibuprofen prevented the carotid body cytokines overexpression, the enhanced hypoxic ventilatory response and the hypertension, but failed to block the enhanced carotid body chemosensory responses. Thus, our studies suggest that the upregulation of TNF-α and IL-1β in the carotid body induced by chronic intermittent hypoxia is linked to oxidative stress, as well as the enhanced carotid body chemosensory responsiveness to hypoxia, but the chemosensory potentiation does not depend on the increased TNF-α and IL-1β levels in the carotid body [18]. However, pro-inflammatory cytokines contribute to enhance the hypoxic ventilatory response and the hypertension induced by ch4onic intermittent hypoxia, suggesting that multiple mechanisms may participate in the cardiorespiratory alterations induced by intermittent hypoxia [18]

Figure 1 shows a diagram of the proposed contribution of the intermittent hypoxic induced potentiation of CB chemosensory hypoxic responsiveness to the hypertension. It is likely that the hypoxic-reoxygenation cycles enhance the CB chemosensitivity to hypoxia, which in turn contributes to elicit a persistent augmented sympathetic neural output.

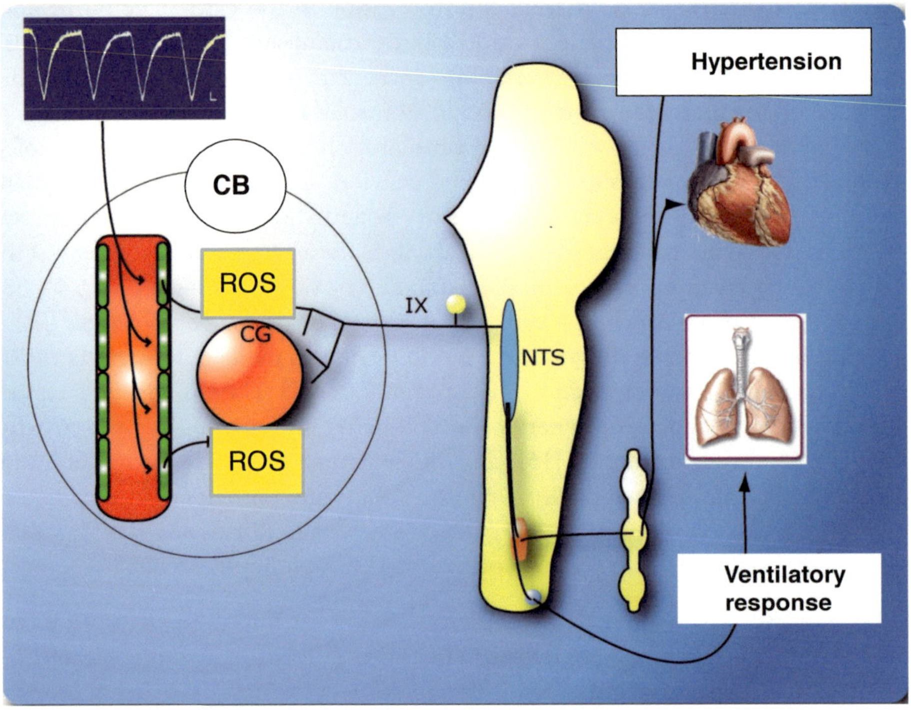

Figure 1. Diagram of the contribution of the carotid body (CB) to the hypertension induced by chronic intermittent hypoxia. ROS, reactive oxygen species. NTS, nucleus of the tractus solitary. CG, chemoreceptor (glomus) cells.

7. Conclusion

OSA patients and animals exposed to chronic intermittent hypoxic shows autonomic alterations and a potentiated carotid body chemosensory responses to hypoxia. The autonomic alterations are characterized by an enhanced sympathetic outflow, a reduction of the efficiency of the baroreflexes sensitivity and alterations of heart rate variability. Indeed, non-invasive spectral analysis of heart rate variability shows a predominance of the sympathetic drive in patients with OSA and animals exposed to intermittent hypoxia. Moreover, direct recordings of muscle nerve sympathetic discharges also showed an increased sympathetic tone and response to hypoxia. Thus, it is likely that the enhanced sympathetic activity along with the reduction of the baroreflex sensitivity could impair heart rate variability and the regulation of vasomotor tone of blood vessels eliciting sustained blood pressure elevation.

Studies performed in OSA patients and animals models exposed to chronic intermittent hypoxia have provide evidence that OSA is associated with enhanced sympathetic activation, mainly attributed to the chronic intermittent hypoxia. The link between the cardiovascular consequences of OSA, including hypertension is multifactorial, most likely related to enhanced sympathetic activity, but also with oxidative stress and systemic inflammation. Understanding how the autonomic dysfunction induced by intermittent hypoxia interacts with metabolic alterations, oxidative stress and inflammation will provide new insights into the pathogenesis of the hypertension associated with OSA. Further basic knowledge will allow proposing and developing new therapeutic strategies to moderate the severity of the cardiovascular alterations induced by OSA.

Acknowledgements

Present work was supported by grant 1100405 from the National Fund for Scientific and Technological Development of Chile (FONDECYT).

Author details

Rodrigo Iturriaga[1*] and Juan Idiaquez[2]

*Address all correspondence to: riturriaga@bio.puc.cl

1 Laboratorio de Neurobiología, Departamento de Fisiología, Facultad de Ciencias Biológicas, Pontificia Universidad Católica de Chile, Santiago, Chile

2 Escuela de Medicina, Universidad de Valparaíso, Valparaíso, Chile

References

[1] Arnardottir ES, Mackiewicz M, Gislason T, Teff KL, Pack AI. Molecular signatures of obstructive sleep apnea in adults: A review and perspective. Sleep 2009; 32: 447-470.

[2] Aydin M, Altin R, Ozeren A, Kart L, Bilge M, Unalacak M. Cardiac autonomic activity in obstructive sleep apnea: time-dependent and spectral analysis of heart rate variability using 24-hour Holter electrocardiograms. Tex Heart Inst J 2004; 31: 132–136.

[3] Baguet JP, Barone-Rochette G, Tamisier R, Levy P, Pépin JL. Mechanisms of cardiac dysfunction in obstructive sleep apnea. Nat Rev Cardiol 2012; 9: 679-688.

[4] Balachandran JS, Bakker JP, Rahangdale S, Yim-Yeh S, Mietus JE, Goldberger AL, Malhotra A. Effect of mild, asymptomatic obstructive sleep apnea on daytime heart rate variability and impedance cardiography measurements. Am J Cardiol 2012; 109, 140–145.

[5] Beebe DW, Gozal D. Obstructive sleep apnea and the prefrontal cortex: towards a comprehensive model linking nocturnal upper airway obstruction to daytime cognitive and behavioral deficits. J Sleep Res 2002; 1: 1-16.

[6] Belozeroff V, Berry RB, Khoo MC. Model-based assessment of autonomic control in obstructive sleep apnea syndrome. Sleep 2003; 26: 65-73.

[7] Biltagi MA, Maguid MA, Ghafar MA, Farid E. Correlation of 8-isoprostane, interleukin-6 and cardiac functions with clinical score in childhood obstructive sleep apnoea. Acta Paediatr 2008; 97: 1397-1405.

[8] Bixler EO, Vgontzas AN, Lin HM, Ten Have T, Leiby BE, Vela-Bueno A, Kales, A. Association of hypertension and sleep-disordered breathing. Arch Intern Med 2000; 160, 2289–2295.

[9] Carlson JT, Hedner J, Elam M, Ejnell, H; Sellgren, J Wallin, BG. Augmented resting sympathetic activity in awake patients with obstructive sleep apnea. Chest 1993; 103: 1763–1768.

[10] Chen L, Einbinder, E, Zhang, Q, Hasday J, Balke, CW. Scharf SM. Oxidative stress and left ventricular function with chronic intermittent hypoxia in rats. Am J Respir Crit Care Med 2005; 172: 915-920.

[11] Cheng JH, Hua CC, Chen NH, Liu YC, Yu CC. Autonomic activity difference during continuous positive airway pressure titration in patients with obstructive sleep apnea/hypopnea syndrome with or without hypertension. Chang Gung Med J 2011; 34: 410–417.

[12] Cistulli PA, Sullivan CE. Pathology of sleep apnea. In: Sleep and Breathing. Saunders NA, Sullivan CE (eds) New York: Marcel Decker. 1994.

[13] Christou IK, Moulas AN, Pastaka C, Gouroulianis KI. Antioxidant capacity in obstructive sleep apnea patients. Sleep Med 2003; 4: 225–228.

[14] Cortelli P, Parchi P, Sforza E, Contin M, Pierangeli G, Barletta G, Lugaresi E. Cardiovascular autonomic dysfunction in normotensive awake subjects with obstructive sleep apnoea syndrome. Clin Auton Res 1994; 4: 57-62.

[15] Del Rio R, Moya EA, Iturriaga R. Carotid body and cardiorespiratory alterations in intermittent hypoxia: the oxidative link. Eur Respir J 2010; 36: 143-150.

[16] Del Rio, R, Moya, EA, Iturriaga R. Differential expression of pro-inflammatory cytokines, endothelin-1 and nitric oxide synthases in the rat carotid body exposed to intermittent hypoxia. Brain Res 2011; 1395: 74-85.

[17] Del Rio R, Moya EA, Muñoz C, Arias P, Court FA, Iturriaga R. Chronic intermittent hypoxia-induced vascular enlargement and VEGF upregulation in the rat carotid body is not prevented by antioxidant treatment. Am J Physiol Lung Cell Mol Physiol. 2011; 301: L702-L711.

[18] Del Rio R, Moya EA, Parga MJ, Madrid C, Iturriaga R. Carotid body inflammation and cardiorespiratory alterations in intermittent hypoxia. Eur Respir J 2012; 39:1492-1500.

[19] Dempsey JA, Veasey SC, Morgan BJ, O'Donnell CP. Pathophysiology of sleep apnea. Physiol Rev. 90:47-112, 2010.

[20] Dick TE, Hsieh YH, Wang N. Prabhakar NR. Acute intermittent hypoxia increases both phrenic and sympathetic nerve activities in the rat. Exp Physiol 2007; 92: 87–97.

[21] Dimsdale J.E, Coy T, Ziegler MG, Ancoli-Israel S, Clausen J. The effect of sleep apnea on plasma and urinary catecholamines. Sleep 1995; 18: 377–381.

[22] Dumitrascu R, Heitmann J, Seeger W, Weissmann N, Schulz R. Obstructive sleep apnea, oxidative stress and cardiovascular disease: lessons from animal studies. hindawi publishing corporation oxidative medicine and cellular longevity, 7 pages http://dx.doi.org/10.1155/2013/234631, 2013.

[23] Eckert DJ, Malhotra A. Pathophysiology of adult obstructive sleep apnea. Proc Am Thorac Soc 2008; 5: 144–153.

[24] Elmasry A, Lindberg E, Hedner J, Janson C, Boman G. Obstructive sleep anoea and urine catecholamines in hypertensive males: a population-based study. Eur Respir J 2002; 19: 511–517.

[25] Feng J, Chen, BY. Cui LY. Carotid body-mediated changes of sympathetic nerve and their relationships with hypertension. Chin Med J 2008; 121: 1732-1735.

[26] Fletcher EC, Lesske J, Behm R, Miller CC, Stauss H, Unger T. Carotid chemoreceptors, systemic blood pressure, and chronic episodic hypoxia mimicking sleep apnea. J Appl Physiol 1992; 72:1978-1984.

[27] Fletcher EC, DeBehnke RD, Lovoi MS, Gorin AB. Undiagnosed sleep apnea in patients with resistant hypertension. Ann Intern Med. 1985;103:190–195.

[28] Garvey JF, Taylor CT. McNicholas WT. Cardiovascular disease in obstructive sleep apnoea syndrome: the role of intermittent hypoxia and inflammation. Eur Respir J 2009; 33: 1195-1205.

[29] Gilmartin GS, Lynch M, Tamisier R, Weiss JW. Chronic intermittent hypoxia in humans during 28 nights results in blood pressure elevation and increased muscle sympathetic nerve activity. Am J Physiol Heart Circ Physiol 2010; 299: H925–H931.

[30] Godoy J, Mellado P, Tapia J, Santín J. Obstructive sleep apnea as an independent stroke risk factor: possible mechanisms. Curr Mol Med 2009; 9 :203-209.

[31] Gonzalez C, Almaraz L, Obeso A. Rigual R. Carotid body chemoreceptors: from natural stimuli to sensory discharges. Physiol Rev 1994; 74 :829-898.

[32] Gonzalez C, Agapito MT, Rocher A, Gonzalez-Martin MC, Vega-Agapito V, Gomez-Niño A, Rigual R, Castañeda J. Obeso, A. Chemoreception in the context of the general biology of ROS. Respir Physiol Neurobiol 2007; 157: 30-44.

[33] Gozal D. Kheirandish-Gozal L.Cardiovascular morbidity in obstructive sleep apnea, oxidative stress, inflammation, and much more. Am J Respir Crit Care Med 2008; 177: 369–375.

[34] Greenberg, HE, Sica, A, Batson, D. Scharf, SM. Chronic intermittent hypoxia increases sympathetic responsiveness to hypoxia and hypercapnia. J Appl Physiol 1999; 86: 298-305.

[35] Hedner J, Grote L, Bonsignore M, McNicholas W, Lavie P, Parati G, Sliwinski P, Barbé F, De Backer W, Escourrou P, Fietze I, Kvamme JA, Lombardi C, Marrone O, Masa JF, Montserrat JM, Penzel T, Pretl M, Riha R, Rodenstein D, Saaresranta T, Schulz R, Tkacova R, Varoneckas G, Vitols A, Vrints H, Zielinski J. The European Sleep Apnoea Database (ESADA): Report from 22 European sleep laboratories. Eur Respir J 2011; 38 :635-642,

[36] Hoy LJ, Emery M, Wedzicha JA, Davison AG, Chew SL, Monson JP, Metcalfe KA. Obstructive sleep apnea presenting as pseudopheochromocytoma: a case report. J Clin Endocrinol Metab 2004; 89: 2033-2038.

[37] Huang J, Lusina S, Xie T, Ji E, Xiang S, Liu Y, Weiss JW. Sympathetic response to chemostimulation in conscious rats exposed to chronic intermittent hypoxia. Respir Physiol Neurobiol. 2009; 166:102-106.

[38] Imadojemu VA, Mawji Z, Kunselman A, Gray KS, Hogeman CS, Euenberger UA. Sympathetic chemoreflex responses in obstructive sleep apnea and effects of continuous positive airway pressure therapy. Chest 2007; 131: 1406–1413.

[39] Iturriaga R. Alcayaga, J. Neurotransmission in the carotid body: transmitters and modulators between glomus cells and petrosal ganglion nerve terminals. Brain Res Rev 2004; 47 :46-53.

[40] Iturriaga R, Del Rio R. Rey S. Cardiovascular and ventilatory acclimatization induced by chronic intermittent hypoxia: A role for the carotid body in the pathophysiology of sleep apnea. Biol Res 2005; 38: 335-340.

[41] Iturriaga, R, Varas, R, Alcayaga J. Electrical and pharmacological properties of petrosal ganglion neurons that innervate the carotid body. Respir Physiol Neurobiol, 2007; 57: 130-139.

[42] Iturriaga R, Moya EA. Del Rio, R. Carotid body potentiation induced by intermittent hypoxia: implications for cardioventilatory changes induced by sleep apnoea. Clin Exp Pharmacol Physiol, 2009: 36: 1197-1204.

[43] Iturriaga R, Del Rio R. Oxidative stress in the carotid body: implications for the cardioventilatory alterations induced by obstructive sleep apnea. In: Oxidative Stress and Diseases. Lushchak VI Gospodaryov DV (eds.). INTECH. Open Access Publisher. www.intechweb.org. 71-86, 2012.

[44] Jelic S, Padeletti M, Kawut SM, Higgins C, Canfield SM, Onat D, Colombo PC, Basner, RC, Factor P, LeJemtel TH. Oxidative stress, and repair capacity of the vascular endothelium in obstructive sleep apnea. Circulation 2008; 117: 2270-2278.

[45] Kales A, Bixler EO, Cadieux RJ, Schneck DW, Shaw LC 3rd, Locke TW, Vela-Bueno A, Soldatos CR. Sleep apnoea in a hypertensive population. Lancet 1984; 2:1005–1008.

[46] Kohler, M. Stradling JR. Mechanisms of vascular damage in obstructive sleep apnea. Nat Rev Cardiol 2010; 7: 677–685.

[47] Kumar GK, Rai V, Sharma SD, Ramakrishnan DP, Peng YJ, Souvannakitti D, Prabhakar NR. Chronic intermittent hypoxia induces hypoxia-evoked catecholamine efflux in adult rat adrenal medulla via oxidative stress. J Physiol 2006; 575: 229-239.

[48] Lai CJ, Yang CCH, Hsu YY, Lin YN, Kuo TBJ. Enhanced sympathetic outflow and decreased baroreflex sensitivity are associated with intermittent hypoxia-induced systemic hypertension in conscious rats. J Appl Physiol 2006; 100: 1974-1982.

[49] Lam SY, Tipoe GL, Liong EC. Fung ML. Chronic hypoxia upregulates the expression and function of proinflammatory cytokines in the rat carotid body. Histochem Cell Biol 2008; 130: 549-659.

[50] Lavie P, Herer P, Hoffstein V. Obstructive sleep apnoea syndrome as a risk factor for hypertension: population study. BMJ 2000; 19: 320: 479-482.

[51] Lavie L. Obstructive sleep apnoea syndrome: an oxidative stress disorder. Sleep Med Rev 2003; 7: 35-51.

[52] Lavie L, Vishnevsky A, Lavie P. Evidence for lipid peroxidation in obstructive sleep apnea. Sleep 2004; 27: 123-128.

[53] Lehnen AM, Leguisamo NM, Casali KR, Schaan BD. Progressive cardiovascular autonomic dysfunction in rats with evolving metabolic syndrome. Auton Neurosci 2013; 176: 64-69.

[54] Lévy P, Pépin JL, Arnaud C, Tamisier R, Borel JC, Dematteis M, Godin-Ribuot D, Ribuot C. Intermittent hypoxia and sleep-disordered breathing: current concepts and perspectives. Eur Respir J 2008; 32:1082–1095.

[55] Levy P, Bonsignore MR, Eckel J. Sleep, sleep-disordered breathing and metabolic consequences. Eur Respir J 2009; 34: 243–260.

[56] Lin M, Liu R, Gozal D, Wead WB, Chapleau MW, Wurster R, Cheng ZJ. Chronic intermittent hypoxia impairs baroreflex control of heart rate but enhances heart rate responses to vagal efferent stimulation in anesthetized mice. Am J Physiol Heart Circ Physiol 2007; 293: 997–1006.

[57] Loredo JS, Clausen JL, Nelesen RA, Ancoli-Israel S, Ziegler MG, Dimsdale JE. Obstructive sleep apnea and hypertension: are peripheral chemoreceptors involved? Med Hypotheses 2011; 56 :17-19.

[58] Marcus NJ, Li YL, Bird CE, Schultz HD, Morgan BJ. Chronic intermittent hypoxia augments chemoreflex control of sympathetic activity: Role of the angiotensin II type 1 receptor. Respir Physiol Neurobiol 2010; 171: 36-45.

[59] Marin JM, Carrizo SJ, Vicente E, Agusti AGN. Long-term cardiovascular outcomes in men with obstructive sleep apnoea-hypopnoea with or without treatment with continuous positive airway pressure: an observational study. The Lancet 2005; 65:1046–1053.

[60] Marin JM, Agusti A, Villar I, Forner M, Nieto D, Carrizo SJ, Barbé F, Vicente E, Wei Y, Nieto FJ, Jelic S. Association between treated and untreated obstructive sleep apnea and risk of hypertension. JAMA 2012; 23: 2169-2176.

[61] Marrone O, Riccobono L, Salvaggio A, Mirabella A, Bonanno A, Bonsignore MR. Catecholamines and blood pressure in obstructive sleep apnea syndrome. Chest 1993; 103:722–727.

[62] McGuire M, Zhang Y, White DP, Ling L. Chronic intermittent hypoxia enhances ventilatory long-term facilitation in awake rats. J Appl Physiol 2003; 95: 1499-1508.

[63] McNicholas WT, Bonsignore MR, the Management Committee of ECAB. Sleep apnoea as an independent risk factor for cardiovascular disease: current evidence, basic mechanisms and research priorities. Eur Respir J 2007; 29: 156–178.

[64] Minoguchi K, Yokoe T, Tazaki T, Minoguchi H, Tanaka A, Oda N, Okada S, Ohta S, Naito H, Adachi M. Increased carotid intima-media thickness and serum inflammatory markers in obstructive sleep apnea. Am J Respir Crit Care Med 2005; 172: 625-630.

[65] Montesano M, Miano S, Paolino MC, Massolo AC, Ianniello F, Forlani M, Villa MP. Autonomic cardiovascular tests in children with obstructive sleep apnea sindrome. Sleep 2010; 33:1349-1355.

[66] Naëgelé B, Thouvard V, Pépin JL, Lévy P, Bonnet C, Perret JE, Pellat J, Feuerstein C. Deficits of cognitive executive functions in patients with sleep apnea syndrome. J Sleep Res Sleep Med 1995; 18: 43-52.

[67] Narkiewicz K, van de Borne PJ, Cooley RL, Dyken ME. Somers VK. Sympathetic activity in obese subjects with and without obstructive sleep apnea. Circulation 1998; 98: 772-776.

[68] Narkiewicz K, van de Borne PJ, Montano N, Dyken ME, Phillips BG, Somers VK. Contribution of tonic chemoreflex activation to sympathetic activity and blood pressure in patients with obstructive sleep apnea. Circulation 1998; 97: 943-945.

[69] Narkiewicz K, Montano, N, Cogliati, C, van de Borne, PJ, Dyken, ME. Somers, VK. Altered cardiovascular variabilityin obstructive sleep apnea. Circulation 1998; 98:1071-1077.

[70] Narkiewicz, K, van de Borne PJ, Pesek CA, Dyken ME, Montano N. Somers, VK. Selective potentiation of peripheral chemoreflex sensitivity in obstructive sleep apnea. Circulation 1999; 99: 1183-1189.

[71] Narkiewicz K, Kato M, Phillips BG, Pesek CA, Davison DE, Somers VK. Nocturnal continuous positive airway pressure decreases daytime sympathetic traffic in obstructive sleep apnea. Circulation 1999; 100: 2332–2335.

[72] Narkiewicz, K, Somers VK. Sympathetic nerve activity in obstructive sleep apnoea. Acta Physiol Scand 2003; 177: 385–390.

[73] Nieto FJ, Young TB, Lind BK, Shahar E, Samet JM, Redline S, D'Agostino RB, Newman AB, Lebowitz MD, Pickering TG. Association of sleep-disordered breathing, sleep apnea, and hypertension in a large community-based study. Sleep Heart Health Study. JAMA 2000; 283:1829-1836.

[74] O'Connor GT, Caffo B, Newman AB, Quan SF, Rapoport DM, Redline S, Resnick HE, Samet J, Shahar E. Prospective study of sleep-disordered breathing and hypertension: the Sleep Heart Health Study. Am J Respir Crit Care Med. 2009; 79:1159-1166.

[75] O'Driscoll DM, Horne RS, Davey MJ, Hope SA, Anderson V, Trinder J, Walker AM, Nixon GM. Increased sympathetic activity in children with obstructive sleep apnea: cardiovascular implications. Sleep Med 2011; 12:483-488.

[76] Ortiz FA, Del Rio R, Ebensperger G, Reyes V, Alcayaga J, Varas R, Iturriaga R. Inhibition of rat carotid body glomus cells TASK-like channels by acute hypoxia is enhanced by chronic intermittent hypoxia. Respir Physiol Neurobiol 2013; 185: 600–607.

[77] Paton JF, Sobotka PA, Fudim M, Engleman ZJ, Hart EC, McBryde FD, Abdala AP, Marina N, Gourine AV, Lobo M, Patel N, Burchell A, Ratcliffe L, Nightingale A. The carotid body as a therapeutic target for the treatment of sympathetically mediated diseases. Hypertension 2013; 61: 5–13.

[78] Parati G, Lombardi C. Narkiewicz K. Sleep apnea: epidemiology, pathophysiology, and relation to cardiovascular risk. Am J Physiol Regul Integr Comp Physiol 2007; 293: 1671-1683.

[79] Pawar A, Nanduri J, Yuan G, Khan SA, Wang N, Kumar GK, Prabhakar NR. Reactive oxygen species-dependent endothelin signaling is required for augmented hypoxic sensory response of the neonatal carotid body by intermittent hypoxia. Am J Physiol Regul Integr Comp Physiol 2009; 296: 735-742.

[80] Pedrosa RP, Drager LF, Gonzaga CC, Sousa MG, De Paula LK, Amaro AC, Amodeo C, Bortolotto LA, Krieger EM, Bradley TD, Lorenzi-Filho G. Obstructive sleep apnea: the most common secondary cause of hypertension associated with resistant hypertension. Hypertension 2011; 58: 811–817.

[81] Peng YJ, Prabhakar NR. Reactive oxygen species in the plasticity of breathing elicited by chronic intermittent hypoxia. J Appl Physiol 2003, 94 :2342-2349.

[82] Peng YJ, Overholt JL, Kline D, Kumar GK, Prabhakar, N.R. Induction of sensory long-term facilitation in the carotid body by intermittent hypoxia: implications for recurrent apneas. Proc Natl Acad Sci USA 2003; 100:10073-10078.

[83] Peng YJ, Nanduri J, Yuan G, Wang N, Deneris E, Pendyala S, Natarajan V, Kumar GK, Prabhakar NR. NADPH oxidase is required for the sensory plasticity of the carotid body by chronic intermittent hypoxia. J Neurosci 2009; 29: 4903-4910.

[84] Peppard PE, Young T, Palta M, Skatrud J. Prospective study of the association between sleep-disordered breathing and hypertension. N Engl J Med 2000; 342:1378–1384.

[85] Prabhakar NR, Peng YJ, Jacono FJ, Kumar GK, Dick TE. Cardiovascular alterations by chronic intermittent hypoxia: importance of carotid body chemoreflexes. Clin Exp Pharmacol Physiol 2005; 32 :447–449.

[86] Reeves SR, Gozal E, Guo SZ, Sachleben LR, Brittian KR, Lipton AJ, Gozal D. Effect of long-term intermittent and sustained hypoxia on hypoxic ventilatory and metabolic responses in the adult rat. J Appl Physiol 2003; 95 :1767-1774.

[87] Rey, S, Del Rio, R, Alcayaga, J. Iturriaga R. Chronic intermittent hypoxia enhances cat chemosensory and ventilatory responses to hypoxia. J Physiol 2004; 560 : 577-586.

[88] Rey S, Iturriaga, R. Endothelins and nitric oxide: Vasoactive modulators of carotid body Chemoreception. Curr Neurovasc Res 2004; 1: 464-473.

[89] Rey S, Del Rio R, Iturriaga R. Contribution of endothelin-1 to the enhanced carotid body chemoreception induced by intermittent hypoxia. Brain Res 2006; 1086: 152-159.

[90] Rey S, Corthorn J, Chacón C, Iturriaga R. Expression and immunolocalization of endothelin peptides and its receptors, ETA and ETB, in the carotid body exposed to chronic intermittent hypoxia. J Histochem Cytochem 2007; 55: 167-174.

[91] Rey S, Tarvainen MP, Karjalainen PA, Iturriaga R. Dynamic time-varying analysis of heart rate and blood pressure variability in cats exposed to short-term chronic intermittent hypoxia. Am J Physiol Regul Integr Comp Physiol 2008; 295 :28-37.

[92] Savransky V, Nanayakkara A, Li J, Bevans S, Smith PL, Rodriguez A, Polotsky VI. Chronic intermittent hypoxia induces atherosclerosis. Am J Respir Crit Care Med. 2007; 175: 1290–1297.

[93] Schultz HD, Li YL, Ding Y. Arterial chemoreceptors and sympathetic nerve activity: implications for hypertension and heart failure. Hypertension 2007; 50: 6-13.

[94] Schulz R, Eisele HJ, Murzabekova G, Weissmann N. Sleep apnea and cardiovascular disease--results from animal studies. Pneumologie 2008; 62:18-22.

[95] Shahar E, Coralyn CW, Whitney W, Redline S, Lee ET, Newman AB, Nieto FJ, O'Connor GT, Boland LL, Schwartzet JE. Sleep-disordered breathing and cardiovascular disease: cross-sectional results of the sleep heart health study. American Journal of Respiratory and Critical Care Medicine 2001; 163: 19–25.

[96] Shiomi T, Guilleminault C, Sasanabe R, Hirota I, Maekawa M, Kobayashi T. Augmented very low frequency component of heart rate variability during obstructive sleep apnea. Sleep 1996; 119: 370-377.

[97] Smith ML, Pacchia CH F. Sleep apnoea and hypertension: Role of chemoreflexes in humans. Exp Physiol 2007; 92: 45-50.

[98] Somers VK, Dyken ME, Clary MP, Abboud FM. Sympathetic neural mechanisms in obstructive sleep apnea. J Clin Invest 1995; 96, 1897–1904.

[99] Somers VK, White DP, Amin R, Abraham WT, Costa F, Culebras A, Daniels S, Floras JS, Hunt CE, Olson LJ, Pickering TG, Russell R, Woo M, Young T. Sleep apnea and cardiovascular disease: An American Heart Association. In collaboration with the National Heart, Lung, and Blood Institute National Center on Sleep Disorders Research NIH. J Am Coll Cardiol 2008; 52: 686-717.

[100] Sukegawa M, Noda A, Sugiura T, Nakata S, Yoshizaki S, Soga T, Yasuda Y, Iwayama N, Nakai S, Koike Y. Assessment of continuous positive airway pressure treatment in obstructive sleep apnea syndrome using 24-hour urinary catecholamines. Clin Cardiol 2005; 28: 519–522

[101] Suzuki YJ, Jain V, Park AM, Day RM. Oxidative stress and oxidant signaling in obstructive sleep apnea and associated cardiovascular diseases. Free Radic Biol Med 2006; 40: 1683-1692.

[102] Svanborg E, Carlsson-Nordlander B, Larsson H, Sachs C, Kaijser L Autonomic nervous system function in patients with primary obstructive sleep apnoea syndrome. Clin Auton Res 1991; 1:125-130.

[103] Tam CS, Wong M, Tam K, Aouad L, Waters KA. The effect of acute intermittent hypercapnic hypoxia treatment on IL-6, TNF-alpha, and CRP levels in piglets. Sleep 2007; 30: 723-727.

[104] Task Force of the European Society of Cardiology and the North American Society of Pacing and Electrophysiology. Heart rate variability. Standards of measurement, physiological interpretation, and clinical use. Eur Heart J 1996; 17: 354-381.

[105] Troncoso-Brindeiro CM, Da Silva AQ, Allahdadi KJ, Youngblood V, Kanagy NL. Reactive oxygen species contribute to sleep apnea-induced hypertension in rats. Am J Physiol Heart Circ Physiol 2007; 293: H2971-2976.

[106] Veale D, Pépin JL, Lévy PA. Autonomic stress tests in obstructive sleep apnea syndrome and snoring. Sleep 1992; 15: 505-513

[107] Williams A, Scharf SM. Obstructive sleep apnea, cardiovascular disease, and inflammation: is NF-kappaB the key? Sleep Breath 2007; 11: 69-76.

[108] Williams AJ, Houston D, Finberg S, Lam C, Kinney JL, Santiago S. Sleep apnea syndrome and essential hypertension. Am J Cardiol 1985; 55: 1019–1022.

[109] Yan B, Soukhova-O'Hare GK, Li L, Lin Y, Gozal D, Wead WB, Wurster RD, Cheng ZJ, Attenuation of heart rate control and neural degeneration in nucleus ambiguus following chronic intermittent hypoxia in young adult Fischer 344 rats. Neurocience 2008; 153: 709-720.

[110] Young T, Palta M, Dempsey J, Skatrud J, Weber S, Badr S. The occurrence of sleep-disordered breathing among middle-aged adults. N Engl J Med 1993; 328: 1230–1235.

[111] Young T, Finn L, Peppard PE, Szklo-Coxe M, Austin D, Nieto FJ, Stubbs R, Hla KM. Sleep disordered breathing and mortality: eighteen-year follow-up of the wisconsin sleep cohort. Sleep 2008; 31:1071-1078.

[112] Ziegler MG, Nelesen R, Mills P, Ancoli-Israel S, Kennedy B, Dimsdale JE. Sleep apnea, norepinephrine-release rate, and daytime hypertension. Sleep 1997; 20: 224-231.

[113] Ziegler MG, Mills PJ, Loredo JS, Ancoli-Israel S, Dimsdale JE. Effect of continuous positive airway pressure and placebo treatment on sympathetic nervous activity in patients with obstructive sleep apnea. Chest 2001; 120:887–893

[114] Zoccal DB, Simms AE, Bonagamba LG, Braga VA, Pickering AE, Paton JF. Machado BH. Increased sympathetic outflow in juvenile rats submitted to chronic intermittent hypoxia correlates with enhanced expiratory activity. J Physiol 2008; 586: 3253-3265.